He
Gave Us a
Valley

Helen Roseveare

InterVarsity Press
Downers Grove
Illinois 60515

Dedicated to Jill,
whose loving friendship made much
of this possible, and
Benj and Basuana, and J. M. and Doctor B.,
and Vera and Abisaya,
and Eugene and Anthony, and so many others
who were deeply involved.

InterVarsity Press is the book-publishing division of Inter-Varsity Christian Fellowship,
a student movement active on campus at hundreds of universities, colleges
and schools of nursing. For information about local and regional activities, write
IVCF, 233 Langdon St., Madison, WI 53703.

Distributed in Canada through InterVarsity Press, 1875 Leslie St., Unit 10,
Don Mills, Ontario M3B 2M5, Canada.

ISBN 0-87784-780-0
Library of Congress Catalog Number: 76-12305

Printed in the United States of America

19	18	17	16	15	14	13	12	11	10	9	8	7	6	5	4
94	93	92	91	90	89	88	87	86	85	84	83	82	81		

Contents

Apologies

Very few names are used throughout this book.
This is not because I think I achieved all this alone.
It is not because I am unaware how deeply indebted I
am to the many who made up the team throughout the
years.
I have not wanted to involve any in the responsibility
for my mistakes, my thought processes and sometimes
faulty deductions.
The blame is mine: the hard work was ours: the glory
is God's alone.

Brief historical résumé

1925 Born at Haileybury, Herts, England.
1931–1944 Primary and secondary school education.
1945 Converted while a medical student at Newnham College, Cambridge.
1953 Sailed to Africa under the auspices of the Worldwide Evangelization Crusade (WEC) to the Belgian Congo. Eighteen months establishing medical services at Ibambi, NE Congo.
1955 Moved 7 miles, to establish WEC medical centre at Nebobongo, comprising:
    100-bed hospital and maternity services;
    leprosy-care centre and children's home;
    48 rural health clinics in immediate vicinity;
    training school for national para-medical workers, that is
        male and female assistant nurses and midwives.
1958 Two years of furlough with further medical training in UK.
1960 Independence: formation of the Republic of Congo.
1964 Rebellion+Simba uprising (civil war): five months' captivity.
1965 Rescued by National Army: one year's furlough in UK.
1966 Returned to Africa under the auspices of WEC to Congo/Zaire, to give seven years' service in an inter-mission (comprising five missions and churches) medical project, at the Evangelical Medical Centre of Nyankunde, NE Zaire, to establish:
    250-bed hospital/maternity complex and leprosy-care centre;
    training college for national para-medical workers;

several regional hospitals and dispensaries;
radio-advisory link-up throughout the medical services;
a 'Flying Doctor Service' through the Missionary Aviation
  Fellowship, to all regional hospitals;
a central supply depot for drugs and equipment.
1973 Home to UK after twenty years of African service.

Was it all worth while?

'But all these things that I once thought very worthwhile –
now I've thrown them all away so that I can put my trust
and hope in Christ alone. Yes, everything else is worthless
when compared with the priceless gain of knowing Christ
Jesus my Lord. I have put aside all else, counting it worth
less than nothing, in order that I can have Christ, and
become one with him, no longer counting on being saved
by being good enough or by obeying God's laws, but by
trusting Christ to save me; for God's way of making us
right with himself depends on faith – counting on Christ
alone. Now I have given up everything else – I have found
it to be the only way really to know Christ and to experience the mighty power that brought him back to life
again, and to find out what it means to suffer and to die
with him.' Philippians 3 : 7–10 (*The Living Bible*).

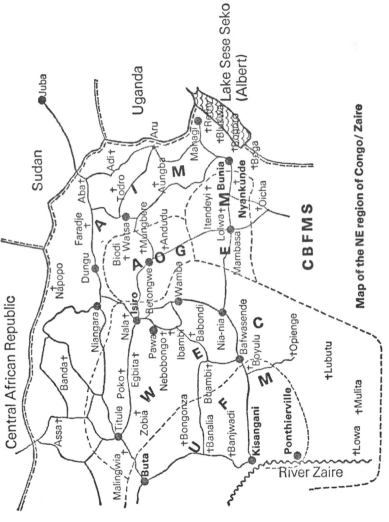

Map of the NE region of Congo / Zaire

Key

—— roads

- - - - rough division between mission areas

+ church/mission centres

● towns

AIM Africa Inland Mission, marking 17 of their church centres, called in Zaire CECA.

AOG Assemblies of God Mission, marking four of their churches, called in Zaire CADZ.

CBFMS Conservative Baptists of North America (not shown on map, working further to the south), called in Zaire CEBK.

EM Emmanuel Mission (Brethren group), showing three assemblies, called in Zaire CAFEZa.

UFM Unevangelized Fields Mission, showing eight of their churches, called in Zaire CEHZ.

WEC Worldwide Evangelization Crusade, showing 13 church centres, called in Zaire CECCA.

Chapter 1 1953-1964
Laying foundations

We chugged steadily across Lake Albert in the small steamer. The mosquitoes were ferocious, and yet unable to imprison me within the butter-muslin walls that surrounded the low bunk in my insufferably hot cabin. I leant on the bulwarks, gazing across the dark ripples, piercing through the night to get my first glimpse of the mountains of what was then the Belgian Congo.

A deep excitement surged through me as the earliest grey of dawn touched the peaks. Was it really possible, after all the years of training and planning and expecting, that at last the true adventure was to begin? I was twenty-eight, with a university degree in general medicine and surgery, from a good, happy home background, stepping out into a new beginning. It was 14 March 1953.

Eight years before, in my first year at university, I had met some Christian students whose quality of life had so challenged me that I was forced to face up to the demands of Christianity. After three months of listening and questioning and watching, various circumstances led to my spending a week at a house-party in London during the Christmas vacation. I turned up at Mount Hermon College to join a gathering of keen Christian girls and young women, training as officers for young people's camps and houseparties the following summer. I just didn't fit: I didn't talk their language. I couldn't understand their spiritual jargon – but I could understand their happiness and friendliness.

I soon found that I enjoyed the orderly Bible study sessions, and I started to read avidly through Paul's letter to the Christians at Rome. The truth began to penetrate my thick skull – it was true! It was no myth. It was no out-dated fairy-tale. This God was *real*, and true, and vital. He cared. He cared for me personally and wanted – fantastic realization! – my friendship. By the end of the week I had capitulated to the clear facts, the obvious reasonableness and the exciting challenge of the gospel. God loved me enough to die for me: would I say thank you? I would and I did. God loved me enough to have a job for me to do in His service: would I sign on? I would and I did.

Perhaps it all seemed a bit of a gamble at the start. I knew so little; but I knew I wanted peace of heart and purpose for living – and no-one else had offered me both. No other religion or political group even hinted at a way of deliverance from sin, a fresh start with a clean slate, a new indwelling power to enable me to achieve the goal. A Christian leader at the house-party wrote a verse in my newly-bought Bible: 'That I may know Christ, and the power of his resurrection, and the fellowship of his sufferings' (Philippians 3: 10). I went to read the verse in its setting that evening, and was tremendously challenged at Paul's dramatic way of stating what I was beginning to feel:

'But what things were gain to me, those I counted loss for Christ. Yea doubtless, and I count all things but loss for the excellency of the knowledge of Christ Jesus my Lord: for whom I have suffered the loss of all things, and do count them but dung, that I may win Christ, and be found in him, not having mine own righteousness, which is of the law, but that which is through the faith of Christ, the righteousness which is of God by faith: that I may know him, and the power of his resurrection, and the fellowship of his sufferings, being made conformable unto his death; if by any means I might attain unto the resurrection of the dead' (Philippians 3: 7–11).

A terrific gamble! What if it didn't pay off? What if it was all an illusion, unreal and untrue? Wasn't it almost too fantastic to believe anyway? Wouldn't one be dubbed a religious fanatic?

Despite the crowding in of such thoughts, I was amazed at myself. Within minutes of a great personal transaction between myself and God, whereby I simply thanked Him for dying for me, believed Him for His forgiveness, and accepted His invitation to serve Him, I had already an ability to laugh at these apparently-specious arguments to put me off. I knew with an unshakable assurance that God was real, that His salvation was true, that I was accepted by Him into His family and His service. God's orderly array of facts in the Bible, plus the consistent witness of the unhypocritical, outright good lives of my new friends, plus now the new ingredient of the persuasiveness of His Spirit in my heart, won the day for me. A great sense of thrill, mingled with a growing sense of privilege, took possession of me.

It took six and a half years to get my medical degree, six months in missionary training centre, six months in Belgium studying French and tropical medicine – and at last, the five-week boat and train journey to East Africa and across half of the great continent to the border of Congo.

Then started eleven extraordinary years of hard work and happiness, mingled with heart-breaks and disillusionments, heights of apparent success alternating with sloughs of despair; yet the net result of all this, judged by the world's standards, was not particularly impressive.

By August 1964 a small 14-acre plot of land in the great Ituri forest of the Congo basin had been turned into a 100-bed hospital and maternity complex with all the necessary ancillary buildings and services. Many of the actual buildings were already there before ever I arrived: many of our team of workmen had been trained by previous missionaries. Subtracting the inherited start from the visible finish, it might seem that we had done very little in those eleven years.

I suppose one hundred patients underwent surgery each year, some of whom would otherwise have died; one hundred young men and women were trained as hospital orderlies and assistant midwives, all of whom would otherwise have remained in relative ignorance; many thousands of babies were born, who would have been born anyway, but with a 50% increase in the chance of survival; many tens of thousands of sick were treated, scores of whom would certainly have died without our help.

But there were moments when I was tempted to ask if this was enough to warrant the enormous outlay of energy and strength.

Individually, and as a team, the medical group involved in the project had learnt a lot over the years. But would that accumulated knowledge justify the expenditure involved and make the whole thing worth while?

The first of many missionary-lessons were taught and learnt right at the start in 1953 at Ibambi. Starting with nothing but an upturned tea-chest, a camp table and a stool, a primus stove and a saucepan, I discovered what it was to be fenced in with difficulties. With no helper, black or white, so much that should have been done to maintain medical standards just proved impossible. Good training told me that a patient with a high fever and chills, painful eyes and profuse sweating was probably suffering from malaria. Treatment in those early days was quinine in a suitable dose according to the weight of the patient, but only after the diagnosis had been confirmed in the laboratory, by seeing the parasite in a blood-smear in the microscope. This microscopic procedure, even in an adequately equipped laboratory, would take a well-trained technician at least five minutes. With fifty or more patients daily showing symptoms of malaria, this would have added over four hours to the day's work. With no electricity, these four hours would have to be worked into the programme during daylight. Yet besides these fifty malarial patients, there were probably fifty others with chest complaints, fifty more with abdominal pain and diarrhoea, and countless more with ulcers and sores. Chest patients needed ten minutes each for history-taking, examination and diagnosis, even without laboratory examination of sputum or radiological examination of lungs. Yet they probably received a cursory glance. Each abdominal sufferer needed careful stool examination besides all other routines, possibly some fifteen minutes each . . .

The day simply wasn't long enough. And so malarial symptoms prompted treatment with quinine, with a quick estimate of weight and no laboratory confirmation. I actually asked God to give me a gift of discernment so that I could pick out the one or two really sick patients with pneumonia or tuberculosis from the line of people with coughs and colds. Similarly, one built up through experience an almost uncanny sense which sorted out the roundworm sufferers from the hookworms, and the amoebic dysentery sufferers from those with bacillary infection – and God overruled.

When I began to realize that over 200 patients were being treated daily, and record cards showed that probably 75% or more were responding immediately to the initial treatment given, I began to see that it was not necessarily a lowering of standards to treat malarial symptoms without laboratory confirmation: rather it was a necessary adaptation to circumstances, with a change of method to achieve the same goal, and with somewhat more realistic hopes of success. These same 200 patients daily, having received something that aided their physical pain to subside, were then much more open to listen to the preaching of the gospel.

Then the first students came. What a motley crew they were! Yokana and Mangadima both from seventh or eighth standard (the equivalent of first or second year at an English secondary school); Mapuno and Bakiogomu and two other lads probably from fourth-grade primary schools, and non-achievers at that; and then Elizabeth Naganimi with no formal education at all, but a bright, keen spirit and a desire to learn and serve. So my second round of difficulties started. I was not a trained teacher; I had no course material; I was going to try to lecture in a mixture of two 'foreign' languages, French and Swahili, neither of which was the first language of student or teacher; and lastly, I was not myself a nurse, and therefore did not know the subject-matter that I hoped to teach!

Again God came to my rescue, and slowly we learnt to overcome this second hurdle. For the first eighteen months of our new training school we wended our way day by day, with moment-by-moment improvisations to meet each immediate need. God taught me to teach as the need arose. There were huge and hideous ulcers every day in the clinic, so I taught how to cleanse them, curette them, treat them and bandage them. A patient came in with burning fever, and so we launched into a lecture on how to use, read and understand a thermometer. In the ward, a post-natal mother developed a high temperature, so we taught the dangers and causes of infection, and how we could prevent as well as treat them. A baby was brought in with broncho-pneumonia, and I demonstrated the use of the stethoscope and how to arrive at a diagnosis. An endless stream of patients, with a seemingly limitless supply of abdominal symptoms, provided us with material to discover the use of the microscope and to learn to recognize every possible species of intestinal parasite.

Students and lecturer learnt together and language very soon ceased to bother us. We created our own course material (aided eventually by the notes of a senior missionary health officer) and went at our own pace. The day of reckoning lay ahead, when we went together for the State final examinations. I for one was intensely nervous, and feared the ditch beyond the hurdle would be our undoing. But the students, in blissful ignorance of what was involved, confident that they knew what I had taught them, and assuming that this must be sufficient, went through with their heads high. By dint of interpreting French questions and Swahili answers, the examiners were eventually convinced that all but one of our group would do good rather than harm, if let loose in a rural dispensary; and we went home rejoicing with six Government-stamped and signed certificates, and six 'medical evangelists' were launched into our new medical service.

There were other difficulties too, on a more personal level, regarding my relationships with my fellow-missionaries. Early on these problems led to loneliness and a sense of insecurity, of not being wanted or welcomed or quite trusted by the fellowship. This, combined with the work-load and consequent inability to take a night off-duty, or to go away for a week-end, brought out in me an irritability and shortness of temper that often caused me considerable loss of sleep. I'd always had a hasty temper, but this had largely been under control for the previous eight years, since my conversion to Christ. Now the hot and angry word would burst out again, before I could control it, and to my shame. Patients who came to the dining-room window while we were at the midday meal would get a sharp word from me to 'go to the dispensary, and not bring your germs to our home' – and a sad look would come to the faces of senior missionaries, who treated every visitor to their home with kindliness and respect.

Evangelist Danga, in charge of the catechists' training course and the workmen's programme at Ibambi, took me to task for this un-Christlike behaviour. 'Don't excuse yourself. Call sin sin, and temper temper. Then face up to the fact that your white skin makes you no different to the rest of us. You need His cleansing and forgiveness, His infilling and indwelling, the same as we do. If you can only show us Doctor Helen, you might as well go home: the people need to see Jesus.'

During my eighteen months at Ibambi I was enormously helped by Danga and the student catechists, by Bakimani and the Bible School students, and by Pastor Ndugu and teams of church elders from various areas of the Ibambi church, to put up two large wards and outbuildings around our dispensary. They taught me to use an axe; to choose the right tree to resist termites and rotting; to select good clean grass and durable fibres for thatching. I learnt how to plan the layout of the building with regard for the prevailing wind, the slope of the roof with regard for the tropical rainfall. I knew how to dig out lime from the right forest streams, and to make whitewash for the walls, not only for its aesthetic look but for its disinfectant value. Together they taught me in the evenings, around the fires, to slice well-dried bamboo and to bind it correctly to make strong, resilient beds, and to weave palm-fronds for roofing and grasses for mats.

Then in 1955, following the graduation day of our first class of students, the medical team was asked to move from Ibambi to Nebobongo, seven miles north. We were asked to take over the care of the maternity and leprosy centres, with the associated orphanage, that Edith Moules had started fifteen years before. Here there were 14 acres of land, sloping down one way or another from a half-mile-long central strip of plateau. Available for immediate use were two brick-built, thatched bungalows for missionaries, similar buildings for maternity care and midwives to the north, and for orphans and widows to the south. A large, unfinished dispensary building half a mile to the west was almost all that was left of the previous thriving colony for the care of leprosy patients, nearly one thousand of whom had been transferred to a Government camp eight miles to the north, or else returned to their forest villages.

So we moved and restarted our medical centre, this time with the outpatients' clinic in the sitting-room, the pharmacy in the dining-room, and the night nurses' room in the guest-room of my new bungalow home. We became instantly aware of our urgent need of other arrangements! The smell and the noise by day, the disturbed hours and the ease of theft by night, made life almost intolerable. New buildings were a must. But how? There was no Bible School with its students, no catechists' school with its workmen, and we did not even have our own church pastor with his team of elders. So who would put up our needed buildings?

I often felt very frustrated by the church arrangements, by which Nebobongo was only an outpost from Ibambi and not a church in its own right. This greatly aggravated the difficulties with regard to buildings. For anything we needed, or for permission to do anything we planned, we had first to apply to Ibambi, which involved a cycle-ride of seven miles of switch-back road in all weathers. This became a constant irritant. The danger of a hot, unguarded retort when asked to do a medical trip to some distant outlying place for one of the missionaries, when I felt (possibly unjustly) that they were unwilling to see our need of help at the medical centre, became more and more real.

We were such a small, insignificant team, yet we were asked to carry such a huge and important burden. At first there were only Florence Stebbing and myself as the missionaries involved, with Agoya our evangelist and his wife Taadi, a group of para-medical auxiliary students and of pupil midwives, and a handful of men, discharged from treatment in the leprosy-care centre during the previous years. None of us had talents or training as builders, plumbers, electricians or mechanics. We learnt by trial and error to make bricks and to fire a kiln: I went to Ibambi to copy in diagram-form their beehive kiln, and then to a local rubber plantation where the Belgian agent had a large, six-firing-hole wet-brick kiln. We discussed the various possibilities, the amounts of firewood necessary for each type, the ease of construction, and, in addition, how to fill in the Government forms needed to authorize the construction as well as to pay the taxes for the firing.

Later again, between clinics and classes, we learnt painfully and slowly the difference between cement and concrete, and how to make each to a consistent quality; how to lay foundations and footings, do corners and bondings, set doors and windows; how to prepare roofing timber and to hoist the triangles and fix the trusses; how to square the corners of the asbestos sheeting and bore the holes for fastening it with nails; how to fix a ridge so that the building did not leak, and the guttering to take advantage of the rainfall.

But it all took time and money; it involved sore hands and blisters; it needed tact and wisdom in handling unskilled labour on nominal wages. And sometimes it was truly hard to see if it was really worth the effort. Through it all, the unskilled labour became at least semi-qualified, to the standard to which the teacher had been able to be taught! This did something for general self-respect and morale, but it also did something in regard to desire and demand for higher wages!

During these years there was the continual problem of responsibilities beyond my training. If the ease with which I responded to the missionary call to service overseas was due in part to my own inherent dread of professional criticism and competition, and the realization that in the heart of the Ituri forest this was unlikely to exist, now there was the horror of responsibility. True, in the medical missionary's life there is unlikely to be much pressure in the rat-race for promotion. On arrival at Nebobongo I became immediately, in the eyes of the national population and the missionary personnel, if not in my own estimation, the senior consultant surgeon, physician, pediatrician and obstetrician. But there was no comrade, no colleague, with whom to discuss cases or to share problems. Always I had to make the decisions of life and death by myself: and I knew only too well how inadequate was my training for this vast responsibility.

In particular, the burden of care for white colleagues weighed on me. Not that I ever wished to treat white any differently from black: far from it! But my African patients did not know enough to be critical. They trusted me unquestioningly and loved me unreservedly. They knew instinctively that by God's grace I would do for them the very best in my limited power, and that this was better for them than no care, or even than witch-doctor care. European patients, however, knew what they wanted, and what they expected: they had home-standards with which to compare our frail and insignificant service.

Then these same Europeans stopped coming to me. Missionaries and tradesmen alike started to make the long, tiresome journey north-east to Dr Kleinsmidt, or the even longer journey south to Dr Becker. And I allowed jealousy to creep in and increase my frustration. How perverse can one be? I feared them when they came, and was hurt when they didn't come! I felt vaguely humiliated by my failure to provide the service that they wanted: and I felt even more wrapped up in a medical loneliness and weariness.

Then in all this whirlwind of activity – construction of new and repair of old buildings; teaching of students and preparing their course material; caring for patients, surgical, medical and obstetric; leading the spiritual as well as the physical life of our family of workmen, students, pupils and children; organizing and supervising some forty-eight rural clinics; ordering and preparing our drugs and medical stores; supervising the work in the small laboratory and down in the leprosy-care centre – in all this the Lord graciously visited our Nebobongo work with revival.

For four years the revival fires had been burning brightly in all the surrounding area, from some 700 or 800 miles south to 100 miles north, from 200 miles west to 100 miles east. Possibly about 100,000 forest villagers had been touched by the fervency of the Christian church in those days. Church services were alive and exciting: no longer slow, monotonous hymns and short, uninteresting sermons. Now everyone sang from their hearts with their faces alight with joy: everyone listened to the preaching of the Word with interest and expectancy. Lives were changed, and ordinary folk lived out what they believed in. Hypocrisy and insincerity were hardly known any longer, especially among the older members of the congregations.

In an ever-changing congregation like ours at Nebobongo, where patients came and went and the student body changed every two years, we needed continuous waves of revival to keep us alight. Joseph Adzanese from the Ibambi Bible School, with his wife Mary, and another couple came to spend ten days with us. Much prayer had been made before and during the convention, and the Lord graciously worked in our hearts. Pupil midwives were first touched: sins were confessed, hearts were cleansed and then filled with joy. Next the blessing spread to the workmen and their families; and finally to the paramedical auxiliary students.

Through the ministry of that convention, and a further ten-day visit to Pastor Ndugu's village, twenty miles away to the east, I also was deeply blessed by the fires of the Holy Spirit. In particular the Lord revealed to me the sin of criticism of others, pride in my own achievements, failure to trust Him in my own inabilities, almost glorying in my frustrations. He showed me again the dangers of over-business, much doing, tireless activity, if it wasn't backed up by prayer. How easily it would all lead to spiritual bankruptcy, and work for work's sake, with no goal of spiritual fruit. In a prolonged period of time apart, alone with God, He filled me again with an intense joy and the deep peace of His abiding presence.

Shortly afterwards I went home to England for furlough and much-needed rest and refreshment, and a period of further medical and surgical practice so as to be better able to cope with the tasks of the future.

Back to Nebobongo in June 1960, as the great day of Congo's Independence dawned. John Mangadima was appointed as Administrative Director of our medical centre, in accordance with the practice of the hour. John had been one of the first group of students who arrived for training in July 1953 and qualified in October 1955. Since then, he had followed two years of training at the Bible School at Ibambi, where he qualified at the close of 1957 as an evangelist and Bible teacher. He returned to Nebobongo at the beginning of 1958 and worked alongside Dr John Harris, another missionary doctor who was in charge at Nebobongo during my period of furlough. Mangadima was proving himself a very able medical auxiliary, a conscientious surgical assistant, a keen and willing administrator: but more important still, from my point of view, a real companion and friend.

Four troubled years of strains and tensions shook the new, young Republic, during which time we sought to consolidate the work of the medical service and to prepare national workers, such as John, for the task of leadership and responsibility. For this, above all else, we required Government recognition for our training programme, and legal certificates in the hands of our qualified workers.

Ever since the inception of the training school for paramedical workers at Nebobongo, we had been applying for this recognition. It was true that, before Independence, our applications had been made with no very great fervour. It had not seemed so essential then, and we had known that the all-Roman Catholic Government was hardly likely to favour a Protestant medical service with official recognition. Through the years of the colonial era, our students had been able to sit their final examinations alongside other students in the region, drawn from similar schools run by the Roman Catholics. The priests had not demurred, as my services as a lady doctor were available to help the nuns in the area as required.

But following Independence our African colleagues started to put pressure on us to make the school 'official'. This was not just as a status symbol, but also because of a growing fear that only para-medical workers with authentic diplomas would ultimately be accepted into the nationalized medical service. Perhaps I was slow. My French was poor; my efforts were spasmodic; my conviction of the rightness of the move was half-hearted. Whatever the reasoning, the recognition had not come. Then a letter came, implying that all un-recognized schools, para-medical as much as secondary, would be closed down. To be accredited was suddenly an urgent necessity.

Fresh letters were written, new forms filled out, different applications put in. Nothing happened! No response was received. John Mangadima pleaded with me to try again. I was fearful of annoying the authorities by my impatience: I was fearful of grieving my team by my apparent indifference. Eventually I re-applied.

One day, as I was using ten spare minutes during the lunch-break to clean out the carburettor of our van, a smart car drove up to my front door. There was Dr de Gott, the local government doctor from Paulis (now Isiro), and with him two strangers, whom he introduced to me as I hastily wiped my hands. They were Dr Trieste, a government inspector from Kinshasa, and Mr Jenkins, a male nurse with the World Health Organization, together responsible for the medical and para-medical teaching programmes throughout the country.

I was shattered. My always-scanty knowledge of the French language seemed to desert me altogether. I was tongue-tied at the awfulness of the situation. This was our legal inspection. On the next hour depended all we had worked for during the last ten years.

Tears stung my eyes. It all seemed so unfair. Why could they not have warned us, sent us word, allowed us time to present ourselves in the best light possible? The telegram to warn us of the date of their arrival arrived two days later, and presumably they never knew that we were completely unprepared.

Dr Trieste almost ignored me, talking rapidly to Dr de Gott about plans they had for developing the three Red Cross hospitals in our area, Pawa, Babondi and Medje. They had just come from Pawa, with its superb ultra-modern buildings and equipment, and excellent laboratory facilities. They were going on from us to see the other two, and also Bafwabaka, the large Roman Catholic centre. They had merely stopped at Nebobongo on their way through, to save petrol. The very way they talked showed that they had never even considered recognizing us.

Their patronizing tone put me on my mettle. We put on the very best show possible. As they went round, I refused to be cowed or defensive, and staff and students responded wonderfully. They spoke up in answer to questions and challenges far better than I dared to hope. I launched out into French explanations, amazed at my own audacity.

True, we did not then get the recognition we so much

coveted, but we were not just written off. We were given two to three years to improve our buildings and to increase our patient/student ratio. In fact the report was remarkably conciliatory, and even complimentary in parts; but as the inspectors were leaving on that traumatic afternoon, I sensed a complete lack of sympathy between the central Government inspector and the local jungle situation.

We did not get recognition. We did not have legal diplomas. There seemed nothing more we could do at the time. What frustration to realize that John Mangadima, capable and mature enough to step into my position, had no official papers to legalize such a move. Legally, he was an 'assistant nurse', as his general education had reached only a certain level. Practically, he was an able houseman to me in surgical and medical services, and a capable assistant in administration and organization.

Not only was I frustrated in my own keen longing to see a national take the lead, but so also was John. He was frustrated in that he had not sufficient outlet for his keen ability, not sufficient stimulus for his acute mind, and particularly not sufficient general knowledge to appreciate that all this was due not to the white man's superiority and unwillingness to hand over, but rather to circumstances of place and timing of birth quite beyond our control. His natural nationalism made him often appear proud; his frustrated leadership ability made him often appear bossy and even offensive to others in the team.

Then suddenly in August 1964 we found ourselves plunged into the horrors of the Simba uprising. The brutality and coarseness of those evil men almost overwhelmed me. Through ten months at Nebobongo they wrought havoc, destroying property, stealing possessions, inflicting cruelties, instilling fear. Shops emptied of all stores. All work ceased and the economy crumbled. Good men were murdered, many others tortured and mutilated. All sense of order and discipline disappeared and anarchy took over. We foreigners were rounded up and taken off to prison, from where we were eventually rescued by the National Army and flown to our various homes. The nationals were hounded and threatened, their homes often burnt and all their possessions looted. Schools were all closed,

24

and even small schoolchildren rounded up to serve as 'Simba reserves', many being killed in battle. Hospitals and dispensaries tried to stagger on, till all supplies were exhausted: and then they too closed down and medical workers, like all others, slipped away into hiding in the great Ituri forest.

Many times in the first ten weeks John, like others, stood by me, and would gladly have given his life if he could have protected me. One day, a car-load of apparently friendly rebel soldiers drove up to my house. John went with me as we crossed the courtyard to them from the school. They asked to be given berets, such as they had seen other rebels wearing. These others had declared that they received them at Nebobongo, but in fact they had stolen them a few days previously from the store of Youth Club uniforms in my home. There were none left, and I said so. Immediately one of them accused me of lying and of refusing to give them what they wanted. He raised his rifle to strike me with the butt-end – and John threw himself between us and took the blow. Eventually we calmed them down with a quip of humour, offering them each a bowl of loganberries and condensed milk and saying that, in English, these were also called 'berries' – and the situation passed.

Another night seventeen wild youths, armed with spears, clubs and crowbars, swarmed into school, demanding our vehicle, the keys and the driver. After much haggling I was eventually forced to drive them to Wamba, 70 miles east, in darkness and rain with no lights or windscreen wipers. Two miles up the road we pulled in at a plantation-factory, to ask for petrol and motor-oil. When a local mechanic brought these, he was then asked to repair the lights and self-starter. I meanwhile stood alone in the dark, conscious that death was very near. I had earlier deliberately disconnected lights, starter and wipers, an act that, when discovered, would be considered blatant sabotage and worthy of instant death. At that moment I became conscious that I was not alone. Turning my head, I found John once again standing beside me, and Joel, a first-year student, with him.

The lights shone out. Shortly afterwards the engine revved up. In a moment of startled silence as the engine cut out, the rebel lieutenant asked if it had been an act of sabotage.

'Assuredly', the mechanic replied: and seventeen enraged youths turned on the three of us, now clearly visible in the full glare of the headlights. The three of us tensed to take the assault, expecting to be instantly in the Lord's presence, when, suddenly, all seventeen were checked, poised in full charge, unable to move a muscle. God had stepped in. It was as though we were surrounded by an invisible barrier of heavenly glory, which blinded our assailants as the midday sun might have done.

'Go on! Kill us – it doesn't matter. We shall go to be with Jesus which is far better. But one day, God will demand our blood at your hands.'

Suddenly, inexplicably, as though they had forgotten our existence, they swung round, loosed from the grip of the paralysing power. Laughing and jeering they piled into the van, forcing the mechanic to drive them away into the night.

And the three of us were left there in the dark and the rain, alone and cold, but *alive*. As we walked home in awestruck silence my heart was deeply moved that these two had stood by me, ready to die if need be, rather than let me face the ordeal alone.

The same happened on the day I finally left Nebobongo. I had been captured several days previously, taken away at night with only the clothes I stood up in. We had been driven to Isiro to be shot, and then had been reprieved, brought back and since held under house-arrest. A senior officer of the rebel troops had visited us and agreed that it was best for the three women missionaries from Nebobongo to stay with those at Ibambi. Then someone had casually remarked that I had not been given time the previous week to 'pack my suitcase' – in the midst of assault and wickedness!

So the rebels had arranged to escort me to Nebobongo to collect whatever I needed to return and live at Ibambi. On arrival, they gave me an hour . . .

The Nebobongo church council gathered at once in my home, and we read from the Bible and had prayer together. Then I handed to one the keys of the office and showed him the books and all the money in hand. Together we agreed to divide it all at once, and to give it out to each member of the 'family', rather than leave it to be stolen by the rebels. I had listed all my 'property' – portable typewriter, ancient bicycle, pressure lamp – and written a letter transferring ownership of each item to one and another member of the team. I talked to Mangadima about drugs and equipment, medical and surgical procedures, and handed him the whole responsibility for the medical service, as acting director in my absence.

Their total silence, tear-filled eyes, pathetic nodding acquiescence in everything I did and said, told its own story. Hearts were being torn open. Each was reeling under the sense of impossible and unwanted burdens of responsibility, and the realization that the one they loved and respected and relied on was actually leaving.

The rebels came back and ordered me to the lorry – plus the hurriedly-stuffed suitcase. And my little adopted daughter Fibi, just ten years old, clung to me, sobbing pathetically.

'Mummy! Mummy! Take me with you! Don't leave me behind again! Please, please, Mummy, take me too!'

My heart ached with a great twisting pain. I hardly dared to look at the child as she clung to my skirt and I pressed her to me. I kissed her tight curls, as my eyes were blinded with tears – and heard a quiet voice beside me:

'Doctor, when Jesus was on the cross, He turned to John and asked him to look after His mother. I'll take your little girl in the same way' – and he gathered Fibi up in his arms and carried her away to his own home. In the moment of my urgent emotional crisis, John had been able to swallow his own grief and the poignancy of his own loneliness and need, and rising above it, to think only of my need.

Then, after we had been driven away, John quietly took over the direction of the medical centre, showing great wisdom as well as courage. Rebel soldiers were everywhere: some were in the wards as patients, one young man with compound fractures of thigh and leg in the surgical ward, and another with severe schistosomiasis in the medical ward. Everything the nurses did was watched and reported. Entering the pharmacy stock-room daily became hazardous, as rebel gangsters always followed, and it needed endless tact and skill to steer them out without their looting the shelves. There seemed little possibility of obtaining any further supplies, and John realized the urgency of preserving all that remained and using it sparingly and without waste: and most certainly, they could not afford loss by looting.

Late one night, silently, alone, alert and watchful, John slipped over to the store and set to work. He divided everything into ten piles – penicillin, aspirins, anti-malarial drugs, vermifuges, sulphonamides and vitamins; syringes and needles, thermometers and bandages, powders and creams. He parcelled up each pile into cartons and plastic bags, listing each article as he did so. Then, glancing cautiously round the deserted courtyard and listening intently for the sound of anyone else awake and prowling, he slipped out with one load, one tenth of all he had.

In the early hours of the morning he woke a village workman and handed him the precious packages. 'Go out now, from the back, in the dark, and bury these somewhere. Tell no-one; don't look inside. Then if rebels demand to know anything, you can honestly say you know nothing. One day I shall ask you for them, but till then, forget about them!'

John quietly repeated this procedure, going every twenty minutes to nine other different workmen. By 4.30 a.m. he had delivered all ten precious burdens, and no-one knew that another had also received a similar task. By daylight everything was buried and all traces covered – and John took a quick hour's sleep before the new day's activities burst upon him.

Through the fifteen ensuing months, roughly every six weeks or so, he visited those ten homes again, one by one, under cover of dark, and recovered his precious stores: and the hospital continued caring for the sick, rebel and civilian alike. Many must have marvelled, and possibly questioned, the apparent ability to continue treatment all that year, with never more than a week's supply of drugs visible! But John kept his secret locked in his heart till after the deliverance by the National Army, and our return with new stocks and supplies.

Other problems faced John and the evangelist Agoya. One was the presence in the nurses' training school of several students from distant parts, who did not know the local tribal languages. Every time rebels raided the hospital and nurses' homes there was danger of a beat-up, as all strangers were suspect of hostile activity. So they arranged for these students to leave and go to stay, two by two, in church homes in nearby villages, away from the main road. But there, another problem arose. Now, instead of the rebels suspecting them, it was the local population who rose against them, treating them as spies as they could not talk their language.

So they were all brought back to Nebobongo, and Agoya and John arranged to care for them themselves, in a hurriedly-constructed dormitory not far from the medical centre, hidden in the local forest land: and there they remained in safety through six months of rebel activity.

At last the National Army arrived and drove out the rebel forces. Nebobongo became an official refugee camp, and troubles even worse than those of the rebel occupation broke upon them. Everyone hiding in the forest was commanded to come out to one of these official camps, so that the National Army could move into the forest to flush out and kill all the rebels. Our small village with facilities for about five hundred under normal conditions was suddenly overrun with several thousand starving refugees – and who was to control the mob?

John and Agoya, with other Nebobongo workmen, did all they could. Every refugee was allocated a 'spot' for sleeping. Church and class-rooms were used, as well as every home and cook-house, and even some of the hospital wards. People were packed in like sardines. Workmen patrolled the food gardens and the avenue of fruit trees, and gave out stores as they could, but nevertheless wholesale destruction and looting commenced on a scale far beyond that of the rebels.

Suddenly the leaders found that the students they had so carefully guarded throughout the rebellion had become the chief of the looters. My lovely home had become a battle-field: 'first come, first served' was the order of the day. The students stole drawers from the sideboard to make suitcases and took the very books from the shelves to make mattresses! Too late the leaders moved in to protect property – there was virtually nothing left to protect!

Then the day came when these same students packed up 'their' belongings to set off on the long trek of 300 miles or more to their homes. National soldiers heard they were setting off, and moved in rapidly. According to the new laws, none could 'walk', that is, travel from one region to another, without the Colonel's permission. The students were therefore taken to the Colonel: one was actually his nephew! Before signing road-passes for them, he demanded that each one should open his suitcase (the drawers of my cupboard closed with padlocks stolen from the pharmacy!).

There was a pause. Soldiers stiffened, alert to the students' hesitation. A menacing silence filled the air.

'Open up,' the Colonel commanded in a cold, quiet voice.

The suitcases were full of stolen property – my clothes and my cutlery, pharmacy drugs and hospital equipment. The punishment for stealing at that time was death.

At that precise moment John cycled up, driven by some inner sense of urgency, and took in at a glance the whole affair. The six students would be shot, including Samuel Yossa, the Colonel's nephew. There was no favouritism, no tribal link now, which could save those who used rebel tactics: they would be wiped out.

John stepped straight through the group and stood before Colonel Yossa.

'Sir,' he spoke with quiet respect, and yet with fearless authority. 'I am responsible for these young men. Let me die in their place.'

A stunned silence. All eyes seemed riveted on John, and then slowly moved to Colonel Yossa. The latter hardly knew John, nor all that was represented in the drama before his eyes, and he turned to his local adjutant for advice.

'This man is our doctor, sir. He is utterly trustworthy, amazingly capable, the medical director of the local hospital. These are students from their training school . . .' His voice trailed away. The situation was beyond him. What could he advise? He'd never heard of anyone offering his life for others. He and most others were maddened by the criminal act of the students, especially after the way John had cared for them through the previous months. So far as he was concerned, they deserved death. But John . . . ? It was impossible to comprehend.

The Colonel gazed steadily at John and marvelled. Yossa

was a godly man, and he deeply admired the quiet courage and devotion of this young man before him.

'Take them away,' he said to John, 'and deal with them as you see fit. Don't let them come near us again.' And he dismissed them all.

John told the students to close their cases and go back to Nebobongo. He was tired and emotionally exhausted. He watched them go, with eyes full of sadness, unable to understand why they hadn't responded to all they had heard of the gospel. The Colonel touched him gently and John turned. The older man held out his hand and they shook hands, one gentleman with another, and the Colonel quietly said: 'God bless you, sir. And thank you.'

As John turned to leave, a soldier gave him six road-passes for the errant students, at a signal from the Colonel; and two days later, the students left Nebobongo to trudge homewards – sobered perhaps, yet rebellious and angry at heart, as their suitcases had been emptied and each filled with two days' food rations only.

From then on, from July 1965 until our arrival in April 1966, John and evangelist Agoya did all they could to reorganize life. There was much to discourage, and at times they were tempted to despair. Chaos and disorder were on all sides. Shattered buildings, roofs riddled with bullet-holes; not a glass window intact; doors and windows and their frames ripped out for firewood. My home was stinking with filth, as the 300 refugees housed there had feared to leave the building during the twelve hours from sunset to sunrise. The refugees had completed the destruction of the primary-school buildings, started by the rebels, smashing forms, desks and blackboards for beds and firewood. Nothing was safe from them.

The committee, organized by John and Agoya, counted up all their resources, everything they had been able to salvage. They brought the books up to date and prepared for a six-month 'period of delay', knowing that they could make no contact with the outside world till far more had been achieved in the way of 'mopping-up' operations. The leaders found they had sufficient funds to allocate a very small token salary to each workman, with which they tried to encourage them to pull themselves together and start work again. Buildings were the prime concern. They checked up on each, evaluating the degree of damage and what would need to be done to make them, at least temporarily, usable. They balanced one against another, and so decided to rip down one to repair the next.

The work proved to be positive therapy against the depression caused by the senseless destruction of the rebellion, and against the disillusionment setting in from the apparent inability of the delivering National Army to do anything for their succour. As the people pulled together to do something of worth, their minds started to tick over and they were slowly persuaded that it was really possible to start all over again. The more they chatted and discussed the pros and cons, the more they came back again and again (so they told us later) to the phrase: 'If only they (*i.e.* the missionaries) come back . . .', and they realized how much we had meant to each other, black and white, just in the even tenor of our everyday lives.

They tackled my home first. The whole long south wall had to be pulled down, the roof shored up, and then all rebuilt, using bricks gathered from the other missionary dwelling which had been destroyed. New window and door frames had to be invented – and the local carpenter Bebesi mysteriously produced a saw, plane and other necessities, suspiciously encrusted with red earth! Up in the roof, a smashed packing-case provided shutters for one window. And so on. Greek merchants had returned to Isiro, 40 miles north, and Aunzo, my cook, was authorized by the group to go and bargain for a roll of cloth, using the tithe of all their meagre monthly allocations – and from this, sheets were made for my bed, curtains put up at my bedroom window, and a cloth laid on the bamboo table that the leprosy patients had laboriously plaited for me.

Taadi, our evangelist's wife, gathered the women together and organized a veritable battery of activities, from a baby crèche to four classes for the primary schoolchildren, from digging, weeding and planting food-gardens to gathering in large quantities of firewood for hospital and homes. Somehow she scrounged one precious chicken from somewhere, and daily they watched it fattening for my welcome feast, for, they reasoned, 'She must come back to us soon!'

32

After the initial flooding with some 3,000 local refugees, these were allowed back to their own villages to start life again: then came the second wave of several hundreds of refugees from 60 to 100 miles in every direction, mostly from the south, desperately seeking food and clothing, housing and security. They were grouped according to tribes, the healthiest in each group being appointed leaders. Each group was assigned a small area down in the largely disused leprosy camp, where they were told to build a new row of dwellings, with cook-houses and toilets, and to cultivate a stretch of land behind each dwelling. Slowly a degree of self-respect and disciplined order was inculcated. There was ever-growing optimism and, I was later told, the frequently-expressed confidence: 'Surely our doctor will come soon!' For me, it was not quite as simple as that.

Chapter 2   January 1966
Am I willing to return?

We had been rescued from captivity on the last day of 1964 and flown home to England. The ordeal over, we had time to rest and recover. By January 1966 the civil war in the republic of Congo/Zaire was virtually at an end. National Army leaders and the major in charge of the mercenary troops were prepared to invite missionaries and traders back to the north-eastern region to assist in the work of rehabilitation, so we were each faced with the question, 'Am I willing to return?'

That there was need for rehabilitation workers was undeniable; the task to be performed was reported as Herculean. Utter destruction and devastation had swept through the vast territory, leaving hundreds of burnt-out villages, derelict schools, plundered hospitals, destroyed shops and thousands of pathetic refugees, homeless and hungry.

Each of us had to weigh up the situation: the need was glaringly obvious, but so also was the almost total lack of material aid to meet that need. The lull in rebel activities was clearly reported, but so also was the sheer impossibility of flushing out every rebel soldier from the thousands of square miles of dense forest. The declared wish of the majority of the population for the return of their 'foreign' friends to help them start life again rang clearly in private letters and public broadcasts, but so also did the definite opposition of a minority group, who felt that the very presence of the foreign missionaries and traders had actually caused some of the worst atrocities of the rebellion.

I looked back as well as forward, as I tried to make the all-important decision. So many memories kept interrupting any orderly line of reasoning, making it almost impossible to reach a sane conclusion. It certainly seemed a crazy thing to do, to go back and start again from the beginning, with nothing except the knowledge that a similar uprising, with similar incidents, could easily happen all over again.

As I tried to review the past thirteen years, the kaleidoscope of experiences that had led up to that final devastating experience became blurred. I could not think beyond the five months' captivity in the hands of the Simba rebels, with their savage brutality and the wanton destruction of all that had seemed so real and worth while, the bestial, heart-breaking, ultimate cruelty of humiliation and rape, of fear and fierce physical pain. The vividness of this final frightful nightmare tended to blind me to all the joy and achievement of the previous eleven years.

I could not just cancel out, as though it had never been, the memory of that awful night of 29 October 1964. I had to learn to live with memory in an understood perspective: I had to learn to accept it as part of the whole before I could possibly face going back to the same place, the same work, the same companions. So I deliberately relived it ...

... the shattering hammering at the double doors of my bungalow home at Nebobongo in the early hours of the morning; the rough, hoarse voice demanding entry in the name of the rebel army; the fear – oh, that dreadful physical torture of fear, with the throat dried and almost closed, the heart strangled and almost stopped, unable to breathe, unable to think. The near panic of senseless unreality. All of 'me' twisted in an agony of terror – and then the calm quiet that seemed to take over like an outside force.

As I nervously clutched a flimsy housecoat over my nightdress, pulling back the bolts of the door, God had seemed very far away and I had felt very, very small and alone. They had swarmed in, rough, uncouth, jeering men in various oddly-assorted garments, smelling of dirt and drink, demanding the man of the house. One separated himself from the rest, in army uniform, leather-belted with holster and cartridges, dark angry eyes, a sense of smouldering hate: clean-shaven, I remember with surprise, with a hard mouth and discoloured teeth. They searched the house; their greedy hands stole what they saw, and their greedy eyes sought me in the glare of their torches. One touched me, and I winced and drew myself inwards. They started to go, stumbling and drunken, laughing and wicked.

The lieutenant had called me back, down the short corridor to my bedroom. 'Go in and . . .' Perhaps I didn't hear: perhaps the hammering in my ears of surging blood and fear made me *think* he said 'undress': he denied it later. I fled out into the dark night, stumbling in the mud, fighting down wild panic as I fell.

'My God, where are You now? Where is Your peace now? Where victory?'

The soldiers came. Naked beams of light stabbed the night, and I was alone. They found me, dragged me to my feet, struck me over head and shoulders, flung me on the ground, kicked me, dragged me to my feet only to strike me again – the sickening, searing pain of a broken tooth, a mouth full of sticky blood, my glasses gone. Beyond sense, numb with horror and unknown fear, driven, dragged, pushed back to my own house – yelled at, insulted, cursed.

'My God, my God, why have You forgotten me, forsaken me?' – the wild cry of a tortured heart – alone, oh, how alone!

Suddenly Christ had been there. No vision, no voice, but His very real presence. A phrase came into my mind, 'led as a lamb to the slaughter', and I saw as it were the events in the garden of Gethsemane, the trial scene, the scourging of Christ, the long march out to Calvary bearing the cross, to the crucifixion. One outstanding fact seemed to dominate the whole: He made no resistance. For my sake, He went as a willing sacrifice. Then, as swiftly, He spoke into my heart: 'They're not fighting you: these blows, all this wickedness, is against Me. All I ask of you is the loan of your body. Will you share with Me one hour in My sufferings for these who need My love through you?'

Two such contradictory reactions possessed my heart in that instance. How could He ask me to *love* these wicked, evil brutes? And yet, how could He, almighty Creator God as He was, condescend to ask me to do Him a favour? Always I was on the asking end, telling Him my needs and expecting Him to give me all I needed: and here He was, presenting me with *His* need and offering me the inestimable privilege of satisfying that need – the loan of my body.

Even as these thoughts chased each other through my dulled mind, the horror of the night continued. I screamed in pain, humiliation, fear – above all, *fear* mingled with pain. Yet, at the same moment, an intense sensation of peace, a strange, deep joy, as He, God, took over from me. Such a mixture of emotions, perhaps it can make no sense to others, yet He was *real* – vital, vibrant, real.

My mind tumbled forward to that day six weeks later, in the convent prison in Wamba, when I had tried to comfort a beautiful young Italian nun, to restore her sanity after repeated raping. She too had given up home and loved ones to come out to Africa to serve God. Maybe I didn't often feel much sympathy for the Roman Catholic cause; maybe we'd had wordy battles on various occasions as we had struggled against each other; and yet, in our suffering, we were one. This young nun had suffered till her mind was torn apart with distress. Her whole reason for living was gone: she had failed to keep her vow of chastity (so she reasoned, unreasonably) and so was eternally damned.

Now we groped towards each other, despite religious and language barriers, to seek the face of the God who *is* love, who *is* peace and power and truth, in the very midst of all that was hate and turmoil, our weakness and their falseness.

'Have you ever stopped to think that the Virgin Mary was called an adulteress by her own friends?'

She recoiled from me as though I'd struck her. Her eyes, dulled before with numb misery, sparked with anger in defence of the holy name that I had degraded.

'Stop!' I pleaded, before she could form a reply. 'Think! Be realistic! It's true. She was pregnant, yet not married. Joseph would say nothing. She just said that it was not his child. What could they all think? Of course they accused her, cold-shouldered her, left her alone and thought the worst of her.'

I paused to let the apparent shock sink into her fuddled

mind. Her eyes pleaded for mercy. I was adding misery to misery. Was I just mocking her, trying to torture her, cashing in on her private suffering?

'Child' (she seemed so young, so vulnerable, so pathetic). 'Mary accepted all that with *joy* for you and me, that the Saviour might be born, the pure, holy Son of God, born of her, Mary, yet conceived by the Holy Ghost. She took the libellous taunts, she bore the stigma, in dignified silence, triumphing over it, because God was in her' – again a long pause, and she slowly let out her breath – 'for you and me.'

Slowly light began to enter the dark eyes. Could this be true?

'Can you take this sin of cruel man against your flesh for His sake, as Mary took the world's condemnation? You haven't sinned: God forbid! It isn't *our* sin. They've sinned against us, yes, but we are only *bodies* for the Saviour to indwell. You haven't lost your purity – rubbish! We never had any anyway: all our self-righteousness is as dirty rags in God's holy sight. But if we have Him who is all pure indwelling us, their wickedness can't touch *Him* or sully His purity.'

She began to talk, to unwind, to tell me of that awful night and the whole nightmare of humiliation. After suffering bitterly at the hands of the coarse soldiers, she had been singled out and taken to the Bishop's Palace. 'But surely he was brutally murdered? Why am I being brought here?' her tired mind had questioned.

The cruel, mocking face of the Colonel of the rebel forces would never leave her. In her Bishop's home, to add insult to injury, the Colonel had claimed her as his wife. All she had, all she held dear, all she understood, was destroyed, shattered, trodden underfoot.

'Why me? Why twice? Why couldn't it have been another?'

Dare one offer her the obvious solace? 'You protected another. Perhaps because you were taken twice, another was not taken once.'

Even in offering this obvious 'comfort', my own heart shrank in horror at the implication, and yet peace and strength came with the wording of the comfort. The God of peace had breathed those words, and they held peace for our hearts. We eyed each other: it was a solemn moment in the very presence of God and slowly both of us felt a great inflowing of immeasurable peace. We touched God, and healing poured into our hearts. That was the first week of December 1964.

I was brought face to face with my own reasoning, my proffered comfort, during the last three days of our captivity, after that bizarre Christmas of 1964, still imprisoned in the convent at Wamba. We had celebrated Christ's birthday despite our prison conditions, with praise and prayer, carols and a crib for our nine children: even with an enormous turkey for lunch! Then the rude interruption of our midday meal: 'Pack. You're being moved.' Curt, to the point.

As always, the fear – the unknown always seemed more evil than the known. Was it just a trap? The first load of nine nuns and four others . . . the second trip with eleven priests and our two protestant men . . . a third trip . . . The waiting, the fierce hoping despite hope, the anxious uncertainty. Then our turn came, at 8.30 p.m. on Sunday night. Rough, crowded, cold, dangerous. That frightful moment when our apparent friend, the Commander of the rebel military police who had protected us during our five weeks' imprisonment in the Wamba convent, left us: and we lurched on into the night, with only an evil lieutenant in charge.

The stop – nowhere, but a house looming out of the darkness. The harsh order to get out . . . and the truck took off into the night, back towards our prison in Wamba. My eyes followed the disappearing roar, while my stomach knotted in a cold sense of despair, a certainty of unutterable evil.

We were ushered into the first room: a settee, a few chairs with no cushions, a table at the other end; windows seemed to be all round and rough guards seemed to be everywhere. We sat crouched on the cement floor, our backs to the wall, watching warily like trapped animals. Three or four younger guards, slightly better dressed, swaggered towards us and we shrank back. The first grabbed at a young woman missionary and Jessie Scholes, wife of our team leader, moved quickly to intercept him. There was an ugly moment as he raised his gun to strike her angrily for interference . . . and the younger woman leapt up, almost offering to go with him, rather than see Jessie struck or hurt.

'She's suffered before,' my coward heart encouraged me.

They dragged another to her feet and took her away. I shrank wretchedly behind the settee and watched her go, with misery and fear in my heart.

'What did you counsel that young nun? O.K. for another, eh, but not for you?' So some voice seemed to taunt me. Still I shrank and prayed to remain hidden from their wicked seeking eyes.

'They're looking round for more prey. Don't forget, everyone left in here, but for you, is so far untouched,' and there seemed to be only one young guard at that moment.

He took me, out into the dark.

Half an hour later I stumbled back into the front room, without looking at anyone, stumbling over dozing forms in the darkness, till I found the settee and threw myself down, wrapped in my own misery. My mind was agonizingly tired. I seemed to be only just holding on to sanity. We were waiting for death, almost all hope of deliverance gone. There didn't seem any point in resistance. Why couldn't they just kill us and be done with it? Why the suffering first? Who would be benefited by all this?

The others weren't back: my heart winced for them and I found solace in praying for them, for their minds, for an ability to accept. Perhaps because I was a doctor, or because my life hadn't been all white in the past, or just because I was me, I had been able to adjust mentally to some extent to this new method of attack against the missionary.

One of the other girls stumbled in . . . minutes ticked by on leaden feet. Another came back. My heart went out to her and my arms drew her down beside me. She sobbed helplessly. We didn't talk. I just held her close to me and loved her, till she quietened and dozed in utter exhaustion. How much her love to protect another had cost her. Oh, those brutes, those brutes, how dared they touch her?

I shook myself from reminiscing and tried to think soberly and constructively. Those five awful months of captivity in

1964 were only a passing episode. I needed to remember honestly the work from 1953 to 1964, and all that God had enabled us to achieve in His service; and then to discover if my part in this work in Congo/Zaire was finished, or if in fact He wanted me back there to help in the mammoth task of reconstruction.

Just what the task might involve was practically impossible to imagine from the comfortable affluence of an English home. Just how extensive had the destruction of the rebellion been? Greek traders, brought to prison in Wamba in December 1964, one month after we had been captured, had reported everything destroyed – buildings, equipment, school and hospital supplies: but we had hoped that they exaggerated. Then the first letters to come out of the war-torn region in August 1965 told us of the loss of all things, and we began to sense a little of what might be the truth.

Doubts gnawed in my heart. Did it really make any sense, starting all over again? The devastating destruction, the enormity of the task of reconstruction, the infinitesimal offering we would have to share: and then what? What had happened once could flare up all over again. What guarantee had we of any lasting peace? What assurance that we wouldn't be wasting our time, that newly-erected buildings wouldn't be pulled down, that newly-stocked hospital pharmacies wouldn't be ransacked?

Were we *really* wanted? How could one begin to assess this in realistic terms? I didn't want to force my services on the Africans if in truth they didn't want me, or would rather be without me. During the years since Independence was declared in June 1960, foreigners had frequently been shown that they were not welcome. Doubtless we deserved much of the treatment we got. For fifty years Africans waited, stood, were ignored and by-passed while Europeans were served immediately with courtesy and given a comfortable chair in pleasant surroundings if a slight delay was unavoidable. It wasn't really surprising that there was a backlog of African hurts to be worked off, by reversing the roles: 'I waited, so now you wait.' Unfortunately the white man had little of the patient forbearance and amazing long-suffering of his African partner, and would often retort or flare up, thereby giving the tormentor great satisfaction at realizing that the needle-prick had found its mark, and so perpetrating the process indefinitely: 'as white, so black.'

True, it was no use being over-influenced by the memory of the coarse shouting of one drunken soldier at a road-block: 'Go back, you dirty white colonialist! Aren't you the cause of all our trouble?' however unnerving it had been, that wild stormy night. Nor must I dwell too much on the treatment I had received at the immigration offices in 1961. A well-dressed, correctly-spoken officer had ignored me all day, leaving me standing outside on the veranda from 9.0 a.m. till 4.0 p.m. My passport lay on his table. He chose to see some twenty or so nationals, all but two of whom had arrived after me, and then told me to 'come back tomorrow'!

Yet these were straws in an anti-colonial wind.

There were of course other straws which blew differently. John Mangadima, as my surgical assistant and close friend, had gone with me, on 13 February 1961, the two-hour weekly journey to Wamba by car, for a day's work at the Government hospital. Just before reaching Wamba we had been flagged down and warned to go home.

'All is chaos. People are fleeing. All the foreigners are being held in prison.'

Puzzled, uncertain, fearful, yet knowing that we must go on to fulfil our medical responsibilities to the patients, over a hundred in number, who were waiting for us, we drove on towards the town. Halted and challenged (and mentally almost demoralized by fear) by a gang of rough soldiers at a makeshift road-block in the suburbs, we were eventually escorted to the authorities. Suddenly everything changed. Smiles, hand-shakes, pleasantness on all sides, and a piece of paper giving me freedom of movement as 'their doctor'. Probably no higher honour could have been offered me at that moment, but the conditions were hardly auspicious for recognizing honour. However, *that* day I was accepted, and wanted, as a doctor to serve them: *that* day the soldiers stood to attention and saluted as we drove past.

Unfortunately I had different treatment only four weeks

later, from the same soldiers, the same authorities, in the same buildings. I was then held prisoner for four fearful hours, because my indicator lights had failed to show I was turning right off a roundabout. The car was brought to a halt by violent gesticulations and wild shoutings. I was ordered out in no un-certain manner and hounded into the police station, accused of no-one-quite-knew-what, pushed around unceremoniously and threatened continuously. I was ultimately fined £20, which I did not have on me. Asking permission for a policeman to escort me to the home of our missionaries for assistance, I was shouted at and ordered not to prevaricate, told to 'pay up or else . . .'. Deciding that silence was the better part of valour, I just stood. Struck and jeered at for not knowing how to answer, becoming muddled with fear and uncertain in my compre-hension of the local French, I just stood.

By then I had been as convinced that I was *not* wanted as, four weeks before, I had vaguely dared to hope that I *was* wanted. So Government officials, soldiers and police had made it pretty clear that, by and large, they no longer wanted the interfering presence of the foreigners.

But what about our own students and medical workers? Was there possibly a different attitude there? I longed to believe that, after the eleven years during which we had lived and worked together, some might be able to overcome the national distrust of the foreigner. Couldn't they believe that we honestly only wanted to help, with no ulterior motive, no paternalism, none of the 'neo-colonial imperialism' about which they were indoctrinated daily from eastern broadcasting stations?

I recalled a particular episode at our Nebobongo medical centre in 1962. John Mangadima, besides being my assistant and friend, was also a strong nationalist, for which I respected him. Sometimes this came over as an 'anti-white' spirit, as on the occasion when the wife of the national regional adminis-trator spent three months in my home, due to difficulties during her first pregnancy. On one of her husband's rare visits to her, John approached him for his advice concerning the scale of wages that the missionaries paid to nurses and workmen. The administrator called a select meeting of local leaders of our medical centre in my sitting-room, and then asked me to attend.

I was frankly nervous, as I had never known if we were wholly within the present law or not, nor whether our interpretation of the law would be acceptable to whoever was in power at any given moment. If the administrator had said that my scale was not acceptable, it could have landed me in enormous difficulties, such as back-paying all hospital employees for two years to Government professional salary-scales, involving as much as £5,000: or a prison sentence to equivalent value, which in Congo at that time might have been for the duration of my life!

We met in strained silence, each avoiding looking at the other. I was scared, but I didn't want to show it. John was half-ashamed, half-belligerent. He loved me and respected me, and he didn't want to hurt me, but nevertheless he wanted to know the truth. He reasoned: 'Everyone knows that the white foreigners are not always straight: they can play with words to forward their own ends.' Not that he blamed us. He really believed that I meant well, but I was white. It wasn't my fault, he knew, but he couldn't ignore it. He felt responsible for the other members of the team who were more easily swayed by my words.

Damaris, the head midwife, was obviously grieved. She wished this confrontation had not occurred. She believed that I'd be hurt and would have done anything to protect me.

Taadi, the evangelist's wife, sat beside me, obviously horrified that anyone could dare to question my word. She believed in me implicitly, and yet she feared some sinister, unknown force.

Each one waited for the other to start. The only one at ease was the administrator. He signalled to John to 'state his case'. John was afraid now, the eyes wary, weighing his words carefully.

'Basically, is it right, under the excuse of a private contract, to pay salaries far below the Government minimum?'

Put like that, it sounded mean, and God knows that I never wanted to be mean. But it was this or nothing, and wasn't this better than nothing? There could be no hospital, no church medical service, if we had to pay Government minimum professional wages. We simply didn't possess the money.

44

'Show me your pay-book,' the administrator ordered John.

Grudgingly he passed it over. He and I were both afraid of being proved wrong, yet neither wanted to hurt the other. The air was tense.

'Really, you are fools,' commented the administrator to the world at large. 'In the world there are two groups of people: those who work for a salary in this life with no preparation for the future, and those who give no thought to the present but are well prepared for the future.' I almost gasped; who would have thought that a Government official could talk like this?

'You have the immense privilege of belonging to the second group: I have the stupidity to belong to the first. And you want to change over?'

John looked decidedly uncomfortable; Taadi was beaming; Damaris smiled her gentle, sad, understanding smile; I breathed a little more easily. The administrator never did answer the actual question. I was to remain for ever in doubt as to whether I was legally right or wrong; but he changed the whole atmosphere and authorized us to continue to find our own solutions.

Had I been able to look into the future and see the tremendous problems of the same kind that lay ahead I might well have decided against returning to start again in 1966. Even without that foreknowledge, there were lurking doubts in my mind as to whether our students would really want us back or not. I knew full well that they desperately wanted classes, teaching, anything we could give them to get life going again. But they were students, educated men and women, not children, and they would be bound to weigh up the cost. Was the apparent price too much to pay? It would mean deliberately subjecting themselves again to what they could only call white domination and paternalism; once again having to say the eternal 'thank you' and to kow-tow to those who seemed always able to give.

I tried to look at the situation dispassionately, to see it with their eyes. I was asking them to trust and believe me, often contrary to their common sense; to believe in my poverty and therefore inability to pay Government wages, when they could see what to them was my blatant affluence. I owned and ran a car: they couldn't. I had curtains at my windows and mats on my floors: they didn't. If I fell sick, I went for medical aid, even if this involved a 500-mile journey by air: all they could afford was a second-hand bicycle. This was all undoubtedly true, however poor I might be in comparison to my counterpart in England, or, more to the point, my African counterpart in Zaire itself. It was true, even if I could comment that I chose carefully and prayerfully how to deploy what little money was at my disposal. My so-called self-sacrifice and generosity were of my own choosing and should not therefore be thought to merit a favourable acceptance and understanding on the students' part. Could I honestly envisage a situation in which I could so get alongside the student body, so listen to their viewpoint and their suggestions, that they would be equally willing to listen to mine, and in mutual trust we could beat out solutions to the many problems that lay ahead? If I wanted to be sure that they trusted me, was I really sure in my own mind, firstly that I was wholly trustworthy, and secondly that I was willing to trust them equally?

As I tried to weigh it all up, it certainly seemed questionable whether we would receive a welcome on returning to serve in the Zaire of 1966, from Government officials, soldiers and police, qualified medical colleagues and co-workers, or from the student body. And yet...

The letters came.

Mangadima, now acting director of the church medical service in our area, wrote and told me of the well-nigh emptied shelves in the pharmacy, and of the endless queues of pathetic refugees and patients seeking medical care that the team were no longer able to supply. He told me that five of the team were working at Nebobongo and four others back at their outlying rural hospitals, so far as he knew, doing what they could with practically nothing. He mentioned that all were working for love of their own people, as no funds were available for salaries. He told me that eleven of the forty-eight students who had been in training when the rebellion disrupted classes had made their way back to Nebobongo, asking if he, John, could not teach them 'till our Doctor comes back'. He ended: 'We don't really expect you to come back after all you suffered from our people, but if God should persuade you to, we will never cease to thank Him, and to love you and care for you as never before.'

Damaris, head midwife at Nebobongo and now in charge of the maternity unit there and the small team of pupil-midwives, also wrote. She told how wonderfully, even miraculously, God had helped her during the months in the forest, both in caring for the orphan babies committed to her charge, protecting them from sickness and starvation, and also in helping women during their confinements in the forest and in the maternity-unit, with little equipment and no help but God's. She told also of the bullet-ridden roof and walls of the maternity-unit, of the smashed windows, of the looted beds and mattresses, of the stolen instruments and equipment. She ended: 'When you come back to us, Doctor, we shall have nothing to offer you but our love, but of that you shall have an unlimited supply!'

Colonel Yossa of the National Army, the uncle of one of our students, wrote to tell of the appalling needs of the people, thousands of refugees needing medical care, thousands of young people needing training. 'If you will come, I personally will do all in my power to ensure your safety, and to assist you in procuring the necessary supplies with which to tackle the task to be done.'

Pastor Ndugu, the spiritual leader of our local church through the eleven years I had served at Ibambi and Nebobongo, a man I had learnt to love and respect, wrote: 'Can you consider returning to us? We need your love and understanding and fellowship; we need your courage and vision and determination; we need your knowledge and wisdom. We have little to give you in exchange, except our love and care, and the peace of God, in the knowledge that you are doing His will.'

Mike Hoare, the commander of the mercenary troops who delivered us from the rebels one year earlier, wrote to others: 'The needs of the people are so overwhelming, that we are prepared to accept responsibility for the safety of the missionaries if they wish to return to start the work of rehabilitation.'

A former student, Cornelius Balani, wrote: 'Don't blame us, Doctor, for all that has happened, but pity us for all we suffer. Come back, please! We are waiting for you expectantly. As God enables us, we will see it never happens again. Please don't remember as important the occasions of student unrest and disobedience: but remember rather the joy and gratitude of those whom you helped to succeed, and know that we others today need you to train us also to serve our people in the medical service.'

Bebesi, carpenter and mason, one of the senior workmen employed by the Nebobongo hospital, wrote briefly but succintly: 'One wall of your home has been blown out and all the roof riddled with machine-gun firing. The other missionaries' home is far worse. So we are stripping it to repair yours. It will be ready for you in two months. I will make shutters for all the windows, as the glass has all gone. I will make you a new bed. You can pay us something when you come, if you want to: but we are happy to work for you without wages, as we love you and want you back.'

Note. The story of these first years, 1953–1966, as summarized in these first two chapters, is told much more fully in two books: *Give me this mountain* by Helen Roseveare (IVP, 1966) and *Daylight must come* by Alan Burgess (Michael Joseph, 1975).

Chapter 3   March 1966
Back in harness

During the three-weeks' journey by boat to Mombasa in March 1966 there was ample time to evaluate my decision to return.

During the year at home, as we had spoken of our African brethren in their suffering, we had built up for ourselves an image of what we passionately wanted to believe. This image had become more real to us than the fading reality of our own sufferings. We accepted the biblical truth that 'in everything God works for good with those who love him', and then we allowed our imagination full play. We pictured the blessing our African co-workers were entering into, in direct proportion to the magnitude of their sufferings.

When their first letters had come, this imagery took even more definite shape and our hearts were thrilled. We glimpsed a preconceived vision and set about preparing for its fulfilment.

Why didn't someone shout at me: 'Pie in the sky!'?

It would have been a good thing if someone had taken me firmly to task, and forced me to listen to sense. Human nature just doesn't work like that. Intense sufferings and emotions do not always produce a total change of personalities.

I had to get down into the valley and look at things a little more realistically: to wake up to life's hard blows and not live in a little world of my own. God did get me to the place, during that sea-voyage to Africa, where I was willing to go back without expecting any dramatic change, willing to accept the difficulties and frustrations that are everyday occurrences in Africa. I should have to learn to see it all with their eyes and understand with their hearts. At home, some had thought we were rather wonderful or courageous or some such adjective, to be going back to Africa again. But our Zairian co-workers weren't likely to think like that: doubtless they were expecting us to return. They had also suffered. Had we not been together? I had had a year's holiday, and hundreds of Christians had given generously to replace all I had lost. Our African friends had just plodded on.

'Why didn't you come sooner?' Would that be their question? Would I be hurt by their reasoning?

Then, too, for a year they had carried on alone: they had managed the finances, repaired the buildings, cared for the sick, been responsible in the pharmacy.

'Will she take it all back from us again?' Would I feel they were obstructing the fulfilment of my vision by their pride, or their obstinacy, or their unreasonableness?

They needed me to raise money for their wages; they needed me to provide the drugs and the equipment, the training and the transport; they needed me as a buffer between themselves and the Government, giving authority to their work.

'Will she do what we want her to do?' – with no question about my vision or my preference, my training or my conception of what I ought to be doing as a missionary. Was I going to resent their reasoning?

During the sea-voyage I became conscious of the old fears again. Why on earth was I going back? Large areas of our region were still in the hands of the rebels. Half a million Africans in the Isiro area had not seen a doctor for eighteen months. Communications were almost at a standstill, and shops were empty of all supplies.

My active imagination painted the scene of long hours and heavy responsibility, not enough drugs and poor co-operation from the Government, uncertainty and insecurity, and I began to think I was a bigger fool than even I had previously reckoned!

Five days in the intense, still heat of Mombasa hardly helped to encourage us! Everyone fights for themselves in a bustling African port or railway station, and noise is an integral part of getting the job done. No good 'thinking white' here. Gathering all our luggage together, re-labelling it for the 1,000-mile journey to the Zaire border, weighing in, clearing customs, loading on to delivery trolleys for port to rail-head, re-checking, paying – all with the rapid calculations needed from one currency to another, and from pound weights to kilograms – in the never-ending roar and rush, heat and haze – all this was a mammoth task, or so it seemed to me!

We faced what seemed like endless delay in unloading the vehicles, endless red-tape in clearing the ton of medical supplies in our van, endless bureaucracy involved in getting permission to drive the 1,000 miles across two African independent states to a third with all the customs formalities, and bearing British licence plates . . . and then on the fifth day I found that the van's battery was missing. My heart sank.

'Possibly the battery has been stowed in the rear of the van, back in England, along with the cab seats, spare wheel, windscreen wipers and other movable parts, to prevent stealing,' I murmured hopefully.

All right, I was allowed to open the vehicle and unload, in the presence of the bonding officer – and also in the presence of the blazing overhead tropical sun! Slowly and laboriously I shifted half a ton of equipment out of the van to the ground, sorted out the needed parts for the journey north-west, and then painstakingly reloaded. There was no battery. There was very nearly complete exhaustion.

The van was sealed and bonded. Four o'clock struck, and all the officials melted into the sticky air except for one agent, who set about to tow me and mine into a bond garage for the night. I climbed into the cab, behind the fast-shut windows, to join the eight hours of captured sunshine in a veritable oven, and I had to struggle to hold back the tears.

Eventually Jessie Scholes and I did escape from the stifling heat of Mombasa and started out on the long climb to the cool of Nairobi, 5,500 ft above sea level. Up again, to 8,000 ft; through the rift valley with its magnificent views; yet again up, to 9,000 ft, and then across undulating hills and down the long slope to Lake Victoria and Kampala in Uganda. More immigration and customs formalities, opening a bank account and doing essential shopping, servicing the van and registering with the British High Commission; and then we said goodbye to Ugandan civilization and set off on the last lap to Zaire.

It was hot and dry. The murram roads threw up clouds of red dust. All along the route smiling villagers and happy schoolchildren waved to us. Herds of wild elephants and wildebeest, wart-hogs and antelope grazed in the surrounding grasslands. So we reached Pakwach, 1,000 miles up-country from Mombasa. This was then the railway terminus, at the source of the Nile.

There to our joy were all our thirty-nine pieces of luggage, but we had no papers with which to claim them – that is, not the *right* pieces of paper! Three hours of typically African haggling and bargaining, spread over a two-hour midday siesta break, eventually secured their release from a highly-amused station-master, by an almost-demented lady-missionary-doctor! Hiring a lorry from a local Indian trader was child's-play in comparison, and thus everything was transported to the Zaire border, still fifty miles ahead of us, up a tremendous escarpment of narrow, twisting rocky road with glorious views.

It was hard driving. At one place we ground to a halt, and I had to search for the book of instructions to discover how to get into low-ratio gears! At another awkward and narrow hairpin bend we encountered the local bus descending the mountainous route, loudly demanding that I reverse to the previous 'passing-point' – which I equally loudly refused to do, demanding my right of way as the ascending vehicle.

'No,' yelled the bus driver, 'I'm the biggest vehicle.'

'Doesn't matter,' I retorted; 'I've a trailer and can't reverse here.'

'I've forty passengers. You must let me through!'

'I'm a doctor: you must concede my right of way!'

Eventually, through sheer inability to reverse down that hill with the trailer, and with dogged pigheadedness, I won! So we continued on through billowing dust to the Ugandan border. Customs formalities were quickly and efficiently completed, and we set off on the eight-mile journey through no-man's-land to the Zaire border.

Here we hit reality head-on. A young American was waiting for us. In fact, he had been patiently waiting for five days! He had the necessary documents to clear all our drugs and equipment, and the van itself, through customs, duty free – but there were no officers when we arrived! After a two-hour wait they rolled up, smell and gait revealing only too clearly where they had been. National Army soldiers accompanied them, carrying rifles, and we quickly realized that we were under a military regime.

It was a strange feeling, this long-anticipated home-coming, so unlike the carefully-rehearsed imagery. It was rough and raw, with coarse language and barely-concealed dislike, drunken and disorderly. It was terribly akin to the rebel occupation – and a tight knot constricted my stomach, and fear welled up in my heart.

'Why have I come back? I must be mad. . . .'

That first night, at the Christian village of Rethy, we were graciously welcomed by missionaries to their bare home, stripped by the rebel occupation. I slept badly and, in nightmare, re-lived the whole horror of those five months of captivity, waking in a sweating panic with one idea only, to get out as soon as I could. I was sure I had made a mistake in coming back. I had thought I'd truly forgotten the suffering. I had thought the fear had died. It hadn't.

I thought I would be wanted, welcomed. I'd built up my own image of what I expected the new relationship to be between national and foreigner, as a result of the suffering – and it just didn't fit.

As we drove from the mountains of Rethy down to the foothills, to Nyankunde, I tried to fix my thoughts on the task ahead of us. Here, at this small Christian village nestling among encircling hills, was the possibility of developing a medical centre and training school for national para-medical workers, and I had been invited to join the team. Dr Becker, a seventy-year-old veteran American surgeon, was already here with two or three European nurses, working in the small thirty-bed hospital that had escaped the ravages of the rebellion.

Dr Becker had worked for over thirty years in Congo, mostly 100 miles to the south at Oicha. Except for his far-superior talent and knowledge, his work there had been much as mine at Nebobongo, with surprisingly similar results, both as regards the painfully unsympathetic inspection by Dr Trieste in 1963, and the traumatic cruelty and disruption caused by the rebellion in 1964. He and his wife had not gone home for furlough, but merely across the border to continue their work in a similar hospital in the south-western region of Uganda. The moment that it was considered 'reasonably safe', they had returned to their labours in war-torn Congo.

I spent one evening with them at Nyankunde, on our way through to our own region. The church was willing to offer us, as a medical team, forty acres of land in the valley next to their own. Already available were two small wards, and two homes for doctors and nurses. In their own valley there was also a fairly small building that had been the outpatients' department, with laboratory, pharmacy and dressing-rooms, before the rebellion. The immediate suggestion was to develop the second valley with a 250-bed hospital and maternity complex, a large block for outpatient clinics and chapel, a building for doctors' consultation-rooms and special ancillary needs, a central laboratory, pharmacy and operative block. The old outpatients' clinic building could perhaps be used as the paramedical training school until new premises could be built.

We talked far into the night. The need was obvious: the means were non-existent. It would have to be team work. Would I ever fit in after years of 'running my own show'?

On Saturday we drove on down from the mountain grasslands into the dense forest jungle and through to Isiro. During that long drive over some 300 miles of rough murram roads, mostly through thick, tropical rain forest, the packed-earth surface cut and criss-crossed with deep gullies from the torrential rains, there were long stretches without a sign of habitation. Then the scattered villages, poor and derelict, seemed to contain only the old, and small children. The many barriers with National Army patrols to control any rebel movements were the only sign of young men. At each of these barriers, we were made very conscious that we were not welcome. The rough drunken soldiers seemed to feel the whole rebellion was, in some mysterious way, our fault.

We approached Isiro, our district town, at 10.0 p.m., tired out. The busy, bustling high street with its gay and noisy shops was deserted and silent, roughly shuttered and desolate.

By now, almost in tears and twisted with fear, I was certain I had made a terrible mistake. Emotionally I just couldn't take it. I told my companions that I'd have to leave.

'O.K., fair enough. But you are our driver for the moment. Take us on the last fifty-mile stretch tomorrow, and we'll make arrangements to get you on the first army plane to fly out next week.' I'd rather face the shame of failure in the relative peace of England, than bask in England's acclaim for courage in the blatant revolution of Zaire. We were not wanted. No-one was calling us brave, or weaving haloes round our heads, or hoisting us up on pedestals. Far from it. We were unwanted: in the way: a nuisance. Hadn't they told us clearly enough to get out and go home, and leave them to cope for themselves without our endless interference?

Next day was Easter Sunday 1966. We drove into our village of Nebobongo, 1,500 miles from the east coast of Africa, at about 8.30 a.m. – and we were mobbed! It was just overwhelming. They were all in church, as we drove up the hill into the village, and they just poured out, Taadi, Damaris, Riotina . . . I couldn't name them all, they came so fast. Then there was John Mangadima, and my twelve-year-old Fibi – we cried a little, among all the hugs and laughter. Nurses, midwives, workmen, house lads, wives, children – all hugs, kisses, hand-shakes, tears, laughter, hand-clapping, singing, praying, rejoicing.

The news had flown down to the leprosy camp, and the patients came up the hill on their stumps, singing and laughing, with bunches of hibiscus and frangipani gripped by their fingerless wrists. Tears ran freely at their abundant love.

On to Ibambi, at about 9.30 a.m., just as the 3,000 local Christians were coming out of morning service. It was quite indescribable. Pastor Ndugu and his wife Tamoma just hugged and kissed me till I felt I would break down altogether. We were nearly torn limb from limb. We shook hands and laughed and wept for a full hour, before being swept back into church for a service of praise and thanksgiving. One has to hear a choir of 3,000 singing from their hearts to believe it possible.

Three thousand faces were radiant, alight with an inner joy and peace.

However, I remember beginning to notice the marks of suffering, the scars on wrists and bodies: then the poverty. The men were in beaten-bark loin-cloths, the women in grass skirts, as they had been fifty years ago when the first missionaries arrived, but as I had never seen them before. There were practically no Bibles or hymn-books – everything had been stolen or destroyed. Some were unbelievably thin, all their ribs sticking out, from months of hunger and near starvation. The lovely church building was pock-marked in the roof, and walls, and floor, from the strafing of machine-gun fire. There was a look of tired strain in many eyes.

Then again, all was swallowed up in the tide of joy, in just being reunited, in knowing the two years of rebellion-suffering were over. The tears did much to wash away the ache and the fear, and eventually blotted out the nightmare and restored peace of heart and mind. Here we were wanted. There was no doubt of that!

They said they had not dared to believe we would ever come back: 'not after all you suffered', they said – and yet their suffering had been so much greater than ours, so long-drawn-out and hopeless. We had gone home from our sufferings and, surrounded by the love and generosity of Christian friends in the homelands, we had been re-equipped and refreshed. They had nowhere to go; this was home. They too lost all, but there were none to replace their loss and re-establish their way of life. Yet they were not morbid, or jealous, or filled with self-pity, just amazed that we were back!

To me, the sense of being wanted was almost stifling in its intensity. They loved us so greatly, I was almost ashamed at how little I deserved it. When we had left them during the captivity, we had distributed all our possessions among them, rather than see the rebels claim everything. We had hardly dared to expect ever to return. Now several Africans brought back to us these gifts to help us settle in again – table and chairs, crockery and cutlery, curtains and blankets – everything they had been able to hide from the devouring hate of the rebels.

In the week that followed, I visited several of the primary schools in the area and talked to children and teachers, and to our educational director. It was truly remarkable how they had carried on. Some groups were gathered in the open air under palm trees, the children doing their writing and sums in the dust of the ground with their fingers. Other groups had put up palm-frond shelters, and children were using bark-slabs as slates, with scrub-thorns as pencils. Masters were teaching all the subjects, including elementary geography, agriculture and hygiene, with no textbooks. 'All I can remember, I tell them, and they repeat it till they've got it by heart,' one young teacher told me.

Hardly anywhere did I see a blackboard or any chalk, desks or forms, exercise books or pencils. There was just *no* equipment. Yet as I entered a school compound, the children would leap to their feet, give their little bow of courtesy with their arms crossed on their naked chests, and then beam at me with happiness. Everywhere they sang, often in four-part harmony. Everywhere they were thrilled to see and welcome a visitor. Nowhere did I hear grumbles or complaints at their poverty – yet the needs were so overwhelming, the task seemed completely impossible.

Sometimes the teachers would unburden their hearts to me. They felt their own Government had forgotten them, passed them by. Who would remind them? They had heard that all those teaching with the old pre independence diploma would be required to give up teaching in a year or so, as only the newer, senior diplomas would be recognized. Who would upgrade them? Or who would replace them? The school buildings everywhere were in terrible disrepair, equipment largely stolen or destroyed, yet there were more children than ever before demanding teaching. Who would rebuild and re-equip the schools?

The educational director of all our primary schools was obviously at his wits' end, dejected and frustrated. Government demands seemed so unrealistic and unsympathetic. The new demands for senior diplomas would cause the inevitable closure of most of our schools. The law binding us to pay the minimum salaries would cause many to be redundant, at a moment when we needed everyone! He had hardly any money available, few qualified staff, no equipment, the buildings all in disrepair; yet the population had gone up by 50% in the previous six years and there were thousands and thousands of children clamouring for teaching. Where should he start? Which way should he turn? Which task should he tackle first?

'Couldn't you please help us?'

They urgently needed someone to train more schoolmasters, taking evening classes, organizing correspondence and vacation courses; to open a secondary school for the crowds of teenagers; to supervise the primary schools, to help sort out all the correspondence relating to Government-subsidized salaries – and I *could* help them. I even longed to help them. Yet...

The medical needs were as great. There were hundreds of sick and no dispensaries, no nurses, no equipment. There were no drugs. The immense difficulties of transport and obtaining import licences were practically insurmountable. Yet I was there among them as their doctor, and they clamoured for help.

The first day after our return we drove our van, the Mobile Hospital Unit, plus trailer, up to Nebobongo, amid enormous enthusiasm. Road-barriers went down before us, happy, smiling guards saluted us: and the Nebo family turned out in force to greet us. How thrilled they were! It was exciting to show them everything – the folded-up stretcher support and the rolled canvas stretcher on wheels; the basin for scrubbing up; the six cans for our stock medicine; cupboards with fitted microscope, laboratory equipment, balance, pharmacy equipment with all the surgical equipment with autoclave and drums; and the forty fitted tins of drugs. The fan, the electric light, the tent extension, the window and fitted mosquito-netting – they looked at and studied and exclaimed over everything. We unpacked and sorted out, put on shelves and filled long-empty bottles from dispensary, maternity, wards and leprosarium, to a continual chorus of excited amazement.

Yet as I went across to do a ward-round, I knew only too well that it was as a drop in a bucket compared to realistic needs. The only thing not in short supply was the patients – thin as rakes, with bloated bellies and spindle legs with great weeping raw areas: tuberculous coughs seemed everywhere, glassy eyes

58

staring out of emaciated sockets. Skin diseases, eye diseases, intestinal diseases. One little three-year-old with cerebral malaria; another with Kwashiokor, weighing only nine pounds. One little boy had an acute cancer of a knee with secondary chest complications. I wrote up treatments from the new stock of medicines just being unloaded from the van to the pharmacy, and knew that, when they ran out, there were no more – nothing but poverty everywhere. No-one had money to pay for treatment; no-one had money to pay a nurse's salary; no-one had money to repair or refurnish the wards. Nothing but poverty: nothing but poverty. The words beat a tattoo in my brain, even in my dreams – mixed with the endless bullet-holes.

I had been down to see the leprosarium, where another welcome party awaited me with flowers and banners. A tremendous effort had been made to repair the large dispensary, but every wall was 'pock-marked' from the machine-gun firing.

I went on a tour of inspection in the maternity block. Everywhere needed paint, but there was none available. Doors were splintered with bullets, and the walls even more pock-marked than in the leprosarium. A great effort had been made to make the roof rainproof, plugging each of the hundreds of bullet-holes. Walls were newly whitewashed, cement floor freshly scrubbed – but this only seemed to accentuate the innumerable bullet-holes. All the ten beds had been destroyed, and the mothers were lying on the floor on raffia mats. The delivery-room had been scrubbed spotless, and a vase of gaudy yellow-orange daisies nodded at me from the delivery table. Two soap boxes on crude legs, covered with butter muslin, housed two minute premature babies – and even here, the mosquito-netting was torn with bullet-holes.

The midwives' homes were clean and tidy, yet leaking badly, roofs strafed by machine-guns. There were no lines of clothes as in the old days, no books, no private possessions – they had lost everything and were bravely starting again.

Back in the hospital, we were called to the operating-room to see a woman who had been struck by a falling tree. I found everything scrubbed and ready for an emergency, a drum freshly sterilized that day with all they had left. There were no scissors, one packet of razor blades: only round-bodied needles and some out-dated cat-gut of rather large dimensions. Looking up as I was scrubbing my hands (in a new basin I had brought that day) I saw one panel of the ceiling had been blown to bits, and two others were pock-marked. Glancing round, every wall showed bullet-wounds, kindly covered with fresh whitewash, but glaring reminders of recent suffering.

The radiographic unit had apparently been totally destroyed: there was no sign of it. The anaesthetic machine had been badly damaged. And everywhere bullet-holes. Poverty and bullet-holes.

They were to be my diet for weeks to come as we fought to overcome both.

Then there were the refugees. They came in droves, endlessly. Mostly they came from the south, shuffling over 50 miles of rough mountainsides, up from the Ituri river basin, over the gold-mine range, and down into the Nepoko river valley. They were destitute and starved. Their pinched faces, bloated bellies, yellowing hair and raw, bleeding feet haunted me for weeks. They told us of hundreds more who never reached us, lying down and dying by the roadside as the final weakness and inability to go on overwhelmed them. And the others just moved on, driven by desperation, unable to mourn, unable even to care.

Day after day, week after week, they came. Who passed the word down the line, that Nebobongo had something to offer? No-one ever knows where hope is born, but their stubborn determination to live, to survive, fanned the flickering hope into a steady beacon of light – and the hundreds became thousands, who trudged relentlessly on. Desolate, hungry, naked, sick. Out of hiding, out of suffering, with *nothing* – no clothes, no food, no tools, no homes.

One month from our arrival back in Zaire, having soaked in a little of the appalling needs everywhere – for schools and teachers, for hospitals and nurses, for refugee centres and supplies – I made my way to Kinshasa, over 1,000 miles away, across the vast jungle basin of central Zaire to the western border of the continent. There, amongst other projects, the Protestant Relief Association managed to get 14 tons of supplies together for me: 60 bales of blankets and clothing, 150 cartons and sacks of dried milk, over 100 sacks of bulgur corn, half a ton of medicines including precious antibiotics, and umpteen sacks of bandages! I managed to buy some £400-worth of blackboard paint and chalk, exercise books and pencils, basic textbooks and maps for one hundred primary-school teachers. Besides which, some hoes, axes, knives and scythes were bought to tackle the great need of rehabilitation.

These were all loaded aboard barges and began the slow journey up-country to Kisangani, where the barges would be unloaded and the supplies transferred to lorries. Then there would be the long, 300-mile journey over fantastically difficult roads. They might conceivably reach Nebobongo in two or three months' time, if all went according to plan!

I flew home to Nebo to continue organizing the distribution of clothing and food that we had been allocated by the local relief organization, encouraged to know that these other 14 tons of supplies were on their way. Agoya and John Mangadima, along with other helpers, were tireless in their care for the hundreds of sick and the thousands of destitute. Immense patience was needed in keeping order among the vast crowds as twice a day they mobbed the 'distribution centre', the small courtyard outside Agoya's home. There, each received a measure of rice or bulgur, a measure of palm oil and one of salt, a bundle of greens and, once a day, some protein addition – dried fish, sardines, corned beef, peanuts or beans.

In the middle of our multitudinous tasks came a sudden, urgent request to go to Isiro to see Colonel Yossa, of the National Army. The week before I had met some Greek traders who had told me they were going to Wamba, where 6,000 refugees had just been liberated by the army. The Greeks had mentioned the destitute state of the refugees through malnutrition and sickness, and also the desolation of the small town, with roofless and windowless homes and broken-down, empty stores.

Now Colonel Yossa wanted to discuss with me the medical needs of these people. He told me that two young Belgian doctors had been in, with a team of national nurses and a supply of medicines, but ... they were frustrated by the enormity of the task and the paucity of their means, and also by the bribery and corruption, the stealing and selling of supplies, even within the team.

The Colonel appealed to me to do something – anything – to help. 'You missionaries have your own way, and you can succeed where we have failed.'

I wavered, and wondered. Could we tackle it?

'There are probably some twelve thousand – they all need you.' My heart lurched. It was sheer lunacy to touch anything so huge.

'Please think about it. We're not ready yet, as we must flush out the rebels from the surrounding jungle and make it safe for you first. But I'll send for you when we're ready!'

Meanwhile, a hundred jobs clamoured for attention. We worked all one morning moving the pharmacy across from the badly-damaged hospital building with its leaking roof, to a room in my house. Every bottle and tin was scrubbed and re-labelled, every drug was counted and listed, a long and messy job, but well worth while when finished. Another missionary spent hours sorting and checking three cartons of second-hand spectacles, labelling each lens and packing them in order. Some workmen were busily putting up four class-rooms for the primary school; another group were cutting poles in the forest for a new home for our evangelist Agoya and his family.

In between other occupations, I squeezed two hours each day to give revision classes to nurses and schoolmasters in Mathematics, French, General Sciences, Geography and Scripture. The aim was to prepare them for the entrance exams to special Government two-year courses, so that they could be upgraded to the new minimal standards.

Ward-rounds were of course a priority. We did all we could with what we had to help some of the tragedy that faced us. Every day, each ward seemed full of pathos, deeply-lined faces, emaciated bodies, skin strung taut across sharp bones, racking coughs, listless eyes. Some particular cases stand out clearly in memory, such as a thin, eight-year-old girl eaten up with a tropical ulcerative disease with great open, weeping sores; a ten-year-old boy with sarcoma of the knee; a four-year-old with cancrum oris, the whole upper gum and lip eaten away back to the nose with a black necrotic ulcer. Always there were pneumonias and cardiac failures, gross anaemias and tuberculosis, every stage of ascites and avitaminosis. The eye diseases had to be seen to be believed. And in the first two months, we finished our precious initial supply of anti-malarial and antibiotic drugs. Where and how to get more was still unanswerable.

Our leprosy patients demanded their share of love and care. During the first few weeks I managed to see them all, old and new, and do fairly thorough examinations and make out new report cards. We had nearly 400 new cases of leprosy in the four years from Independence to the Rebellion: but now, following the deliverance, we were flooded with almost another 400 new cases among the refugees.

I was given an overwhelming reception. Everywhere was spotlessly clean – pharmacy, treatment centre, examination-room, waiting-hall, hospital ward – tables and cloths, report cards and medicine bottles. Outside, the courtyard was swept clean, and even flower-beds weeded and tended. The half-mile-long road through their village was bordered with pineapples, and neat, well-cared-for food-gardens with peanuts, rice, manioc and plantains behind each small home. These people might be sick, with fingers and toes mutilated, their feet and hands often ulcerated and stumped, but they were happy and hard-working.

Throughout this period of two or three weeks, we kept hearing reports that the people at Wamba were in great need, with many, many dying of starvation and illness – and I wrote a note to Colonel Yossa to say that I would go for a week in mid-July, if medicines could be procured. I suggested he should get an American army transport plane loaded with relief supplies from Kinshasa to Isiro, and we would see to fair distribution at Wamba.

I had to go to Kisangani on another urgent errand, but I talked there also of the urgent need at Wamba for relief work. Suddenly things started to happen. Bill Gilvear of Relief Agency talked it over with 'Big Bill', an American in charge of a private air service, put at Zaire's disposal during that difficult period. I was bull-dozed into preparing a report of what I thought I could handle (clothing and blankets and food for

10,000, and medical supplies for treating at least one quarter of them). These were made out in six copies, in French and Swahili, stamped and signed, and flown to the American Embassy. I thereupon became terrified at what I had offered to do and, not for the first time, wondered why on earth I had become so involved.

Radio messages started snapping over the thousand miles from Kisangani to Kinshasa. Our request was reiterated and confirmed. Eventually it reached the President's ears. Everything seemed to be whirring into top-gear activity.

Then a message came that Kinshasa would provide drugs, but we must collect our own relief goods. So I set out on a crazy walk round Kisangani, from store to store, from Greek trader to Indian trader, from Protestant Relief warehouse to Catholic Relief warehouse: and slowly, by sheer stubborn determination, I coerced them into supplying me with over 10 tons of corn, oats, bulgur, wheat, milk, soya bean oil, plus clothing and blankets.

Then the 15-ton transport plane flew in from Kinshasa, and I hurried out on to the tarmac to check the bulk supply of drugs, only to find the plane was empty. 'The General of the National Army is sorry, but your order is too big.'

Another almost frenzied rush around town. The pilot gave me only two hours to collect what I could before he must take off, if he was to make Isiro in daylight. The Spanish doctor at the Government hospital gave me all he dared; the newly-opening medical faculty of the University shared all they had with us; Dr Barlovitz, a private doctor in town, supplied a huge crate from his own clinic; both pharmacies in the high street fell to my impassioned pleas; and what with twelve more bales of clothes and blankets, two more tons of milk and soya bean oil, we filled that plane in those precious two hours!

I tried to get my breath back on the one-hour flight to Isiro, and started to plan for the task ahead. Lists of urgent needs flashed through my mind: camping equipment – beds, blankets, kitchenware, food, tableware, chairs, tables. Lists of people I could ask to help me – Colin and Ina Buckley from Isiro, Agnes Chansler from Ibambi, a junior nurse from Nebobongo, my cook and the Wamba pastor would all need to go.

When we reached Isiro, life really began to move fast. We faced deluging rain and miles of slippery mud. At one point on a steep, narrow hill, with deep water-gullies each side, two lorries were already stuck! I ploughed out in wellington boots, measured the gap, and weighed up the possibility of getting through, when the Egyptian driver of the second lorry offered to drive mine through in exchange for a lift into town – an offer I accepted gratefully!

Packed up, with trailer behind, we set off on the hundred miles to Wamba on the Saturday afternoon. As we crossed over an almost non-existent bridge into the Wamba territory, we were struck with the desolation – broken-down houses, unkempt gardens, deserted villages submerged in a wilderness of weeds.

Perhaps notes from my diary of the next seven days will give the best impression of that fantastic week.

Saturday 16 July. Arrived at the post at dusk, we went to report to the officer in charge. The first shops we passed, the transport house, the Government offices, the post office were all completely roofless and destroyed. The prison still stood in its sordid square. Along the one main road, all the gardens had been cleared and tidied: buildings were mostly inhabited by army, and in fair condition: till we reached the shops. One, two, three, four – the main shopping centre – utterly destroyed. What pathetic waste! We found the two white mercenary officers sitting with our Greek friends, Mr Mitsingas and Mr Dimitriou. We chatted amiably, and told them we wished to stay at the Mission for a week.

Up at the Mission, we went straight to Daisy Kingdon's home – in fairly good condition. It had been the 'Simba' headquarters and office, and was now being used as National Army government office. Various families in possession but they moved out for us. We swept and cleaned, and slowly moved in. Certainly rough living! None of the original furniture. Few odd tables and rickety chairs, and doorless, shelfless, cupboards, and *dirt*! Windows and doors largely without hinges or fixtures – but we soon had a pot of tea boiling and felt ready for anything.

Back again to see the Greek merchants and 'borrow' buckets, bowls, mugs, etc. for the work of distribution, and then to the Catholic Mission to invite them to take part with us in the distribution.

Sunday 17 July. Three church services and fellowship with some 500 church members. Prepared for tomorrow. A team of 50 helpers are all ready, each knowing their part. Chairs, tables, cards, date-stamps and ink-pads, bowls, buckets, mugs, spoons – all have been checked and distributed to the helpers. Bamboo 'fences' have been erected to guide the crowd where we want them. 200 vials of penicillin have been prepared, and 16 syringes and 144 needles sterilized. Between us nearly 5,000 report cards have been serially numbered.

Monday 18 July. A grand day! We heard them coming at 5.30 a.m. – and in no time some 400 were queueing up. All the helpers were soon in place, each with their necessary equipment. Primus stove burning, with saucepans of syringes and needles: bowls of Quaker oats with mugs for giving out: bottles of iron tablets: and so on. At eight o'clock we 'opened the doors', and in half an hour we had near anarchy! About a thousand people scrambled to get in first! At that moment, the mercenary lieutenant and three Congolese soldiers drove up in a jeep – and in ten minutes, perfect order!

By midday, we were through for today. 2,600 people had passed through, of whom 400 received medical cards, 70 of these being for severe malnutrition (almost 3% of those we saw). Ten of these malnutrition cases were deeply pathetic to see. One woman with six children – all emaciated, with swollen feet, sores, yellowing skin and hair. We gave what treatment we could, of supplementary protein and vitamins and also penicillin injections.

It is interesting that only 16% of the people were in acute need of medical aid: probably 50% were suffering from diarrhoea, mainly due to malnutrition, but doubtless also due to intestinal worms and dysentery. Ninety-four people had severe eye infections. We expect to see much more sickness tomorrow, now that the news will have spread around.

During the afternoon, a note came up from the African head-nurse at the Government hospital – a woman obviously needing a Caesarian section operation. I went down at 4.0 p.m. and we did it together – with the one and only blunt scalpel, four artery forceps, no sponge-holders, no gauze, no general anaesthetic – but all went well. We had no masks or gowns, just gloves: and no nail brushes. What poverty! But we had lots of faith and goodwill, and God helped us.

Tuesday 19 July. A thick, damp mist as light slowly broke through this morning, and the queue had started. By 9.0 a.m. there were about 2,000 to the left of the church porch, all with tickets from yesterday, and about the same number to the right, stretching as far as the eye could see, across the compound, all along the football field, out and across the main road, and down through the gardens opposite. And still they came! Everything was very orderly, with two soldiers to help us outside and fifty-six church elders helping with the distribution inside.

In all today, 5,176 people went through, representing 2,032 families. Of these, 1,015 received medical help, about 20%. The malnutrition cases were truly pathetic. Skin and bones, oedema and ulcers, thrush in their mouths and glazed eyes. We gave each of them milk, every two to three hours – they just *grabbed* it, and cried for more. They were starved and desperate.

At midday, two more truck loads of supplies arrived – milk, oil, corn and clothing. In the afternoon, some essential shopping, plus pulling a molar tooth for the Greek trader! In the evening, we erected more barriers to direct the crowd for tomorrow's task of distributing clothes – trousers and a shirt for each man, a piece of cloth and a blanket for the children, and a dress for each woman.

Wednesday 20 July. What a day! We're all almost worn out! By 6.0 a.m. the battle was on, in a cold damp mist, a queue stretching away to the far boundary of the compound. When the doors were opened, the flood released! In seven hours, 4,630 had been through, including 650 sick, receiving penicillin, worm treatment, eye ointment, iron tablets and milk. Then we prepared for the 'first-timers': a vast and ever-increasing crowd. In four hours, we had let 2,238 people through, and treated a further 328 sick, bringing today's total to 6,868 people served with oats, corn, iron tablets and each receiving a garment, and 978 sick helped medically.

From 5.0 to 6.0 p.m. it *poured* with rain and I was soaked, walking up and down the line, keeping order, enforcing discipline, acting as a barrier against gate-crashers. Many 'Simbas' joined the lines, but I'm afraid I hauled them out. I just couldn't agree to giving them food and clothing after all the suffering they have inflicted on others. The last two hours, we had the car headlights on the queue: the extension light on the exit: and two pressure lamps and five storm lanterns in the hall.

On Thursday, all the population is expected to clean and weed the town and surrounding area. I've been to see the Congolese lieutenant this evening, to ask permission for our sixty assistants to have a day's holiday, and also for the 1,400 people on penicillin treatment to be allowed to come up for their injections. He agreed amicably.

Thursday 21 July. I suppose this amazing week will end one day! This morning we did some 600 injections, treated over 100 Kwashiokor children, tried to keep order among the thousands who hoped for food and clothing distribution, encouraged the soldiers with a good deal of humour to keep calm and not to throw their weight about!

This evening, we have given out full food rations to the 116 'helpers' and their wives and families – about 550 altogether: and clothes! What a tremendous job, fitting every little boy and girl, woman and man, with a suitable garment. It has taken a *long* time, but we had to do it after dark, to avoid attracting another vast crowd. Giving out clothes attracts more than even penicillin, and far more than food!

Friday 23 July. By 6.0 a.m. there were vast queues in every direction, and a great wave of unbelieving disappointment when I broke the news that we could serve no newcomers, only those with tickets in their hands. Once again at the door a green date-stamp on their medical cards, a purple date-stamp on their food cards: divided into four files, to receive a mug of Quaker oats and a mug of soya bean oil: passing by the medical workers for penicillin injections, eye ointment or bandages: handing in their tickets at the exit, where I collected all food cards, and any medical cards with five consecutive dates, and returned other medical cards dated for a final injection tomorrow.

Everything moved *fast*. Keeping the count was quite exhausting work. At 9.30 a.m. Ina Buckley brought me a mug of coffee and two sandwiches. As I took a bite, a passing child grabbed the sandwich from my hand and absolutely shovelled it into his own mouth, and then looked at me pleadingly for the other. I have never seen such desperate hunger – I could do nothing but hand the child the second, and watch it disappear in a few wild, famished gulps. Oh, if only folk could see the pathetic need!

We were finished by 11.0 a.m. – every flake of oats had gone: every drop of milk was finished. 4,885 people had passed through and each received some help at least. Tidying up, sorting out, writing reports – and an early lunch.

The continual noise and crowds, pathos and needs, have been very wearying and we are all feeling that a week is all we can manage at a stretch.

Saturday 23 July. Our time at Wamba has ended.

In some ways, a success story: over ten thousand refugees helped with food and clothing and medical care. Yet this was one small group, perhaps one per cent of all that needed doing. Already the Government was talking of plans to repeat this week in some fifty other needy areas, but they have not the personnel or the supplies to implement their plans. And we realized that we had hardly scratched the surface of the tremendous and appalling needs.

Chapter 4   May 1966
How could I be so foolhardy?

In the welter of need, each of the returned missionaries and of the church elders sought to find his own priorities. It wasn't easy, in the middle of everything, to see the wood for the trees. Why were we in Zaire? And what were we meant to be doing, individually and as a group?

After three weeks at Nebobongo and in the area, soaking in the needs of schoolchildren, patients and refugees, I went back to Nyankunde to discuss and pray with Dr Becker, as to what we should tackle first.

Dr Becker had already made his own decision: that all interested missionary societies and church congregations should create a new medical team, and that together we should build one good, central hospital for the vast region, where Africans could be cared for in body, soul and spirit, to the highest possible standards.

Would I join him?

For a week Dr Becker had to be away from Nyankunde, working at the mountain hospital of Rethy. So I went with him and we worked together, doing ward-rounds, general surgery, outpatient clinics and special eye clinics day after day. All the time we discussed the various possibilities of this tentative plan. At one moment it seemed possible that we might approach the Government and offer to take over one of their hospitals, as at Bunia, and run it for them. But as we discussed it, all the impracticalities became so abundantly clear that we dismissed the idea. We became more and more certain that what was needed was a Christian centre, where Christlike behaviour as well as teaching formed the essential basis of all the activities. We needed the right to appoint, discipline and dismiss staff, in order to maintain spiritual and medical standards. We needed the right to select students for our training college from our respective church secondary schools.

As we discussed and worked together, a definite over-all plan began to form itself in our hearts and minds. Our vast region was some 500 miles square, a great basin of tropical rain-forest, bordered to the east by the mountain range on the foot-hills of which Nyankunde was situated. If we could develop a 250-bed hospital at the Centre with facilities for 1,000 out-patients daily, and first-class medical and surgical, obstetric and pediatric care, all this could support a training school for twenty-four students annually in a three-year course. Young men would be trained as medical auxiliaries to run rural hospitals and dispensaries, and young women as auxiliary mid-wives to run the accompanying maternity units. We envisaged a network of a possible dozen regional hospitals, in the care of European nurses at first, helped by Nyankunde school graduates, until these could be upgraded and able to take over the leadership: and each of these regional hospitals to be surrounded by some ten or a dozen rural dispensaries.

Our imagination ran on, and saw every one of these medical-health centres served by radio-contact to the Centre at Nyankunde, so that any nurse or auxiliary, national or foreigner, could discuss difficult cases directly with a doctor and receive all possible aid from the Centre. Then we realized the essential need of a small plane and pilot, to link up every outpost with the Centre, with half-mile long airstrips to be cut out of the forest at each dispensary and hospital.

Quickly our minds moved on to the problem of medicines and equipment. We would need a central pharmacy at Nyankunde to undertake all the problems of import licences customs duties, transport, reception, checking, stocking, sorting. From here each outlying hospital and dispensary could order its monthly needs.

The next step in our thinking was easy: one doctor from the

Centre should be freed from other responsibilities each week to fly to one of the regional hospitals to do a week of medical oversight and surgical care, to help the nurse in charge with administrative problems, and to distribute the needed drugs and equipment. Thus the benefit of our work at the Medical Centre at Nyankunde would be spread over the largest possible area, and give the maximum help to as many as possible of the five million inhabitants.

Throughout our discussions, my mind kept flicking back to the need of a training school, to train Africans to the highest possible standards of nursing and medical care for their patients, as well as in diagnostic principles and practice; to train them for the job that most needed doing, in all the out-lying regional hospitals and dispensaries. Already I was men-tally listing the subjects to be taught, how many hours of each to each class, methods for combining practical with theoretical training, report sheets to record the progress of each student. I was picturing class-rooms and laboratory, nursing arts' demon-stration room and assembly-hall, offices and record filing. I could visualize dining-hall and dormitories, uniforms and en-trance exams. Each evening after prayers, as I went to bed, I scribbled all my thoughts down, covering reams of paper. I drew up lists of suggestions, lists of possible students, lists of proposed courses practical and theoretical.

My heart and mind were caught! Already I was visualizing the future years, seeing graduates from our training centre serving all over the region, not merely as skilled medical workers, but above all as medical evangelists. With my whole being I believed in the rightness and necessity of teaching and training others to do my job. To me, this was virtually an obli-gation laid upon me, in exchange for permission to live in Africa. My principal desire was to train medical auxiliaries whose prime objective was to show Christ to their patients, not only in preaching, but through the standard of their medical practice and the loving care given to each individual.

Back at Nyankunde the following week, we paced over the 40 acres (20 hectares) of land that we were being offered for the Medical Centre. Dr Becker had already commenced building, and had already in his heart and mind a vision of the whole. We were situated in the bowl of two hills. Around the hills, as we looked up the valley, were to be the homes of the medical staff. The school and playing-field, dormitories and dining-hall, would be in the centre. Then spreading out down the slope below, away to the north, the hospital, with laboratory and pharmacy, X-ray and maternity, operating theatre and intensive care unit. Twin wards were to be built on either side of a central corridor: and finally the administrative block and offices, outpatient hall, clinics and chapel.

There was room already assigned for a 'self-help' village, for distant patients who did not require hospitalization: also for a small tuberculosis village, leprosy-care centre, and psychiatric wards: for laundry, garages and workshops.

So I returned to Nebobongo again, churning over all the exciting new possibilities, and wondering how I could 'sell' my vision to the Ibambi church elders. I needed the local church to be with me in this project, or I felt sure it would fail. I wanted them to release me from my immediate task at Nebobongo, of helping children, patients and refugees in our own church area, to go far away – 350 miles of rough roads, two days' driving – to start a school. It all sounded a little lame, put like that. Would it sound like running away from overwhelming, obvious, pressing need, to hide myself in a small, comfortable spot doing a small, enjoyable job? How could I convince them that ultimately it was for their own good? If I can train some of their sons and daughters, I told myself, to obtain the new Government medical auxiliary diploma, they would then have workers for several hospitals and dispensaries, instead of just me alone at Nebobongo.

I knew this was true, but I also knew it didn't sound convincing. A bird in the hand is worth two in the bush. A doctor now seeing to their multitudinous needs at Nebo seemed much more worth while than the vague possibility that in a few years' time they might have some half-qualified help. 'They are never going to be doctors, are they?' I could hear them asking.

Throughout the long, tiring fight against mud and ruts, during nineteen hours of journeying, including being pushed and tugged out of two giant-sized mud-holes, my mind ploughed on at the problem. Was it right? Could it work? Would the others agree? Could I 'sell' it to my WEC colleagues, nationals and missionaries, by promising to visit them twice a year, to supervise our medical services? The awfulness of those 350 miles appalled me, and then I would have to add a possible further 1,000 miles' circuit to visit our three northern, central and southern hospitals and their many dependent dispensaries. The road surfaces were all deteriorating rapidly; some bridges were dangerously near to collapse; many of the hills were practically impassable after rain. My heart failed at the prospect of regular trips.

Back at Nebobongo, I met the church elders and nurses to tell them of all our deliberations at Nyankunde, and the proposals for the new school. They were stunned. I had only just got back to them; they had no other doctor; how could I ask them to agree? Even the suggested twice-yearly visits raised little enthusiasm. The prospect of a monthly visit by a doctor/ surgeon by plane certainly fired them to set to and cut an airstrip out of the surrounding forest, in order to make this dream a reality. The fantastically high fees proposed for students at Nyankunde Nurses' School were terribly discouraging to them in their abject poverty, and I vowed in my heart to procure scholarships from somewhere.

For two days I prayed over this with them, and we sought God's mind. Then together we went to Ibambi to meet the church council, and again I rehearsed carefully all our proposals. Their discouragement was hard to accept. They just couldn't bear to think of my going away again, and no-one to replace me. I dared not even encourage them overmuch by promising visits from the 'Flying Doctor Service'. Our small hospital at Nebobongo suddenly seemed so utterly primitive, after I had visited various medical centres of the other Missions, with their electricity generators, running water, permanent buildings and huge crowds of outpatients. I had become ashamed of our little medical centre. Had I been so immersed in my own inadequacy that I had fatalistically accepted poverty and inadequate buildings and supplies? I seemed to have done so little for them – and yet I reminded myself that many hundreds had been healed in body and spirit through the work at Nebobongo during the previous twelve years.

Another two days of prayer, and we discussed the problem from all aspects. On the second day, they received a letter from a missionary who had been the director of our secondary school. We all knew that, during the year of the Rebellion, he had gone to work for another church area. Now they were anxiously awaiting his return to re-open the school. He was their one hope for the thousands of children needing secondary education, and also for the training of national teachers for the hundreds of primary schools. But his letter came to tell of the overwhelming needs down south, with over 1,000 boys finishing sixth-form primary school that summer, and only one teacher available to accept them into secondary school. Therefore he was asking the church to allow him to stay down in the south for a further two-year period. Our church council was stunned. Their own overwhelming need was so appallingly apparent that they simply couldn't believe that their one secondary-school director was not returning. They felt deserted.

And there was I, doing virtually the same thing. How desperately we needed reinforcements in the way of schoolteachers, doctors, nurses and secretaries, as well as mechanics, builders, electricians, radio technicians, air pilots and general administrators. Where were the workers to fill all the gaps?

Eventually, by the end of the week, albeit grudgingly, the council agreed to wish me God-speed, and allowed me to go ahead with the new vision that had started to burn in my bones. I left immediately on the long journey to Kinshasa, the capital of Zaire, to lay the plans before the central Government and to secure their rubber-stamp on our blueprints.

The country was, of course, still emerging from the torture of the two years of internal strife and bloodshed, so ordinary methods of communications and transport were almost non-existent. I hitch-hiked the 1,500 miles in an army transport plane, noisy, cold, uncomfortable, but free! Then started three weeks of foot-slogging and dogged perseverance, to seek the right people for our cause, and to persuade them to be sufficiently interested for a sufficiently long time to grant us some sort of pledge of their co-operation and assistance.

At the same time as I was presenting our plans for developing a Medical Service centred at Nyankunde, I was also endeavouring to procure residence visas in the passports of the five WEC missionaries. What a thankless task! We had applied for these over seven months previously, and had not heard a word since then. The Christian travel agency which handled these affairs for us was non-committal and discouraging. I was not the only one seeking a visa, it appeared! And no-one really knew how to tackle the task, or hurry officialdom.

A taxi-ride two miles up the main boulevard; a vast flight of steps, a wide corridor with many doors; folks hurrying here and there, doing nothing apparently but carrying huge portmanteaux; others holding up the walls as they discussed at length, in high-sounding French, why they should not do what their superior had ordered, and why he had no right to order them to do it anyway. Down a narrow flight of stone steps, to Chancery. It was truly Dickensian, even in the elaborate, outdated vocabulary. A large, elderly African came forward and I explained my need.

I was nervous and anxious not to offend or to appear in any way critical of their right to make me wait seven months. Yet I was eager to state the case clearly, even if apologetically, trusting they would then serve me. He retired to his desk and began searching in the only file in it, among some twelve sets of application papers and photographs. Eventually he sorted out our five and came back with them. Again I went through all our reasons for applying for permanent visas. At last he motioned me to leave *that* room, pass through a door in the corridor, and re-enter the same room by the next door, to the same counter but farther along.

Here I explained to the *same* man all that I had already told him twice. After a short delay he led me into another, larger room, almost empty except for four large desks around the edge and Congolese officials perched on high stools behind them, through an opening to the second half of this hall, with a further four desks, only here the officials sat on chairs!

I was led to one senior official and introduced to him. I

repeated my story, clutching the five sets of application papers with their photos. He took our passports and examined our expired visitor-permits. As he had not fully understood me, I repeated again the circumstances of our arrival in Zaire during January and March. He went and discussed the matter at length with another official. They returned together, and I recited *again* the tale of my distress! Conferring together, they decided to send me to 'Immigration' – 'just over there, by the monument'. He gave me a note of introduction to 'Immigration', asking that I be treated with courtesy and alacrity as I had already waited seven months.

I set off to walk 'just over there, by the monument' and took a quarter of an hour to reach the monument, and a further five minutes to discover the office. I waited in a queue, and showed my letter of introduction. I moved to another queue at a window and repeated the performance. From there I moved up two rooms and joined another queue. They passed me on to an office at the 'back', but the official there was obviously not pleased to be found, just twenty minutes before closing-time. The argument grew fairly heated, but all he assured me was that I was 'unofficial' and must become 'official'.

A Belgian technical adviser offered to drive me back to the Ministry of Foreign Affairs, guided me back to Chancery, introduced me to the same large African to whom I had already told my story three times, who escorted me back to the high official who had sent me 'unofficially' to Immigration. He accepted all my precious sets of applications and photos, promised to 'process' them the same afternoon, and told me to go to Immigration the next morning, by which time I would find that I was truly 'official' – but by then I had no letter of introduction! I felt I had moved a distinct step forward, but subsequent conversation with others who had shuttled for months between Chancery and Immigration brought me a large measure of doubt as to whether I would ever see our forms again, officially or unofficially.

So, next day, to Immigration – no news, but forcefully told not to go again! Back to Chancery, where I drew a blank: just 'Come again at 2.0 p.m.'.

Back again that afternoon, and that time I actually saw our

five names on a list that had been sent to Immigration for in-dexing. When (and if!) that list returned, I could collect our visas. Chancery said hopefully that they might be ready in three days: everyone else prophesied they might be ready next year!

Three days later, in the torturing heat, I presented myself once again at the Ministry for Foreign Affairs, looking for our visas. From there I was once more directed the mile to the Immigration Office. But no luck! The applications had passed through the first office, to another – but who would stir them out of there, no-one seemed to know!

A week later the search was still on, but by then I had got an able assistant, Jessi Nkoma, a very accomplished, educated African. Under his pressures the application papers were eventually found and transferred to the right office, and the man in charge promised them for the next day.

So Jessi went back for me the next morning, but was told to return in the afternoon!

That evening, he burst into the home where I was staying, waving my passport triumphantly in the air, duly stamped with the required resident visa! But . . . not the other four! To-morrow. . . .'

Meanwhile our main business was to gain recognition for the Nyankunde project for a medical centre and training school. During my first week in the great city I had made my way to the Ministry of Public Health to see the Secretary General, Mr Nandu. While I was waiting for him in the ante-room, Dr Trieste, the inspector of all medical and para-medical educa-tion in Congo/Zaire, came in. Recognizing me from that trau-matic inspection at Nebobongo three years previously, he was gracious and even courteous, and arranged to see me in his office at the end of the following week, when I could present him with our proposed school programme.

Mr Nandu arrived and received me in audience most en-thusiastically. He listened patiently and keenly to all my ex-planations and to our three main requests, namely:

    a. recognition for the new school, immediately;

    b. a five-year period for the war-stricken north-eastern

region, during which candidates might be accepted for para-medical education with less general secondary education than demanded elsewhere;

c. upgrading and recognition for our older para-medical assistant nurses, trained between 1950 and 1964.

It seemed obvious that I was not the first doctor to approach him about these burning questions. He felt that if I presented all this to Dr Trieste immediately, before the meeting of ministers the coming week, there was a very good chance of the first two points being granted at once. This would then allow us to bring in the older assistant nurses, who showed capabilities of being upgraded, during the five-year extension programme.

I was really amazed at how quickly he had assimilated all that I had presented, especially as I myself was becoming increasingly tired, with the strain of talking and thinking in and listening to French all day, and keeping exactly to the appropriate points with each different official to whom I was presented.

When I eventually reached Dr Trieste's office I was even more tired, from ten days' foot-slogging to get the necessary documents signed for presentation to the Ministry, and not a little discouraged by it all. Dr Trieste walked in ten minutes late for our appointment, nailed me with two sharp, piercing eyes, and demanded brusquely: 'What do you want?' There were no preliminaries, no introductions, none of the courtesy of our earlier encounter, and a hint of: 'I've no time for you – two minutes at the most. I'm a busy man. . . .'

'All I want is . . .' – a moment's hesitation – '*sympathy*' I added quickly, remembering that inspection at Nebobongo three years ago, when he had declared our training school unsuited for Government recognition, despite our ten years of sweated labour.

I think he was taken aback momentarily by my reply. There was a pause; then he actually smiled!

I leapt in and outlined hurriedly the whole desperate situation in the war-torn north-east; and, refusing to be daunted by my obvious inability to get the subjunctive tense or right concords into my utterly ungrammatical French, I rushed on into the plan forming in our minds to meet those needs.

He listened, at first idly, doodling on his blotting-paper; then more intently, eventually becoming caught up by my enthusiasm into jotting down notes. *Then* things started happening.

'O.K. How concrete are your plans? Have you a time-table for how you can achieve all this? Building plans? Curricula?'

I gulped – gazed – and pledged anything he wanted!

'Give me the use of a typewriter, paper, carbons and a pen, and I'll produce all you want.'

'Go ahead then – use my desk. I've a meeting with the Minister in ten minutes. I'll tell him that I want to see him again tomorrow with your proposals.'

He left, and I started to work, from 10 a.m. through to almost midnight. I drew plans and drawings of proposed buildings; I worked out time-tables for a four-year course both for students and for staff; I made out a decidedly optimistic budget with no suggestion of where the funds would come from. Then I worked on proposed record cards and diplomas, methods of organization and suggestions how to bend the present law to allow for the recovery of the north-eastern region over a five-year period. It all seemed a wild gamble of imagination! I nearly got cold feet as I realized I had no authority from our team at Nyankunde to commit them so completely.

At midday I managed to contact Dr Becker through the Missionary Aviation Fellowship radio network, and got his permission to go ahead. I'd no idea how much he then understood of what I was promising to do in his name! But he was wholly in the project and prepared to back me all the way.

By midnight I had left the completed file on Dr Trieste's desk, drawn up as an eight-year project to establish the training school, with buildings up to the required Government standards, curricula following the suggested Government scheme, and all the staff necessary to implement it. And I fell into bed in a daze of doubt. How could I be so foolhardy as to think I could ever achieve it? But God . . . !

For two weeks I had to wait for a word from Dr Trieste, but at last the word came. He then took me on a wild tour of various departments, from one end of the city to the other, seeing secretaries, functionaries, administrators, and eventually the Under-

Secretary to the Minister. As we went we gathered up papers, documents, forms; course material, models, books for our non-existent library (though most of this material was for a course either junior or senior to our proposed one: there just wasn't any available material for what we wished to teach); and an enormous quantity of enthusiasm, goodwill and encouragement.

'Go ahead with your plan. We'll send inspectors up as soon as we can,' and with this I had to be content. No written word, no signature, not even a firm promise, but I inferred that recognition would follow inspection if we could complete our side of the bargain in the stipulated time.

And so back to Bunia to give a full report to all the team at Nyankunde; to start work on preparing entrance examinations, and building plans for the first phase of the new training college.

A week later I set out for Nebobongo, despite many transport problems. I managed to hitch-hike a lift on a cargo flight to Kisangani with two and a half tons of *pork*! I had been waiting two days at Bunia for a regular flight that never came, when I saw a DC3 come in and begin unloading cargo. I went quickly through the waiting-hall and out on to the tarmac, to see if I could possibly get a ride. A Greek was loading pig carcases. A Belgian gentleman also wanted a place. Two passengers would be allowed by the pilot if two carcases were unloaded. Much heat ensued, and argument in many languages. 'Impossible', the Greek roared, working out his financial loss through such an arrangement.

I just stood quietly by, with my suitcase, in the shadow of the wing of the plane, and waited.

Fiercer arguments – greater heat – still he shouted: 'Impossible!'

They all went off to the office and I heard the altercation continuing. Someone came out to the plane; two carcases were taken off, carried back to the hall and weighed, and my heart rose.

More shouting, gesticulating, fury; the Greek returned, and the two carcases were thrown back on. Still I waited.

Then it all occurred again . . and the pilot and co-pilot

arrived, obviously furious. 'Get in quickly: go up to the cockpit and sit in the co-pilot's seat – make yourself conspicuous!' Totally baffled by the last part, I did as I was told. The pilot revved the engines up, we taxied out, and climbed up into the air – when I was told to make my way back to a seat amongst the pigs! I gathered the pilot was mad with the trader for thinking a miserable pig's carcase more important than a lady doctor! He then made it clear that he took me in his seat at his expense, and the old trader could care for his own conscience!

Our students who had been in training before the rebellion sat their entrance exams for Nyankunde. Papers came in from eleven other centres and schools, and I spent a day marking and sorting, finally selecting four classes of twelve students each for the first year at Nyankunde.

The fantastic activities of the week among the refugees at Wamba came as a surprising interlude in all our other activities, including steady preparation to leave Nebobongo to start a new life at Nyankunde. As the date to move grew nearer, all sorts of alarming rumours also grew. Kinshasa radio reported violent uprising between Katangese troops with mercenaries and the National Army, involving the death of Colonel Chache. Colonel Yossa went from Isiro to Kisangani to verify reports, and found himself landed in prison. General Mulamba was expected in Kisangani from Kinshasa, and the air was full of speculations.

I met with the Greek traders in Isiro and discussed how all this might involve us. It seemed probable that there had been a planned 'coup', as the Katangese troops had all left our region some weeks before and there seemed no obvious reason for their return. Some were frankly optimistic, other hopelessly pessimistic. When the evening news stated that the 500 whites in Kisangani were 'safe', it sent a shudder through me, to hear again the sort of language we had heard all through the Rebellion. In Isiro, there were two or three days when officers were having difficulty in maintaining calm and order among the excitable troops. The major had even wanted to blow up the bridges on the Kisangani road and cut down trees as roadblocks. As excitement and rumour mounted, all the soldiers were made to lay down their arms. We missionaries were requested to stay at Ibambi, despite the rising tensions, as the sub-lieutenant said that our presence would give assurance and exert calm in the explosive atmosphere: he promised to send an armed escort should we need to be evacuated in a hurry.

But when 26 July, the day for leaving, dawned, we all felt that it was right for me to go ahead with our programme and to start the journey to Nyankunde. Our Land Rover and trailer were loaded to capacity. Pastor Danga of Wamba and my friend, Jacqueline van Bever, were in the cab with me, and behind, like sardines, were John Mangadima, his elder brother Naundimi, Benjamin, my house lad, and Cornelius Balani, a senior nurse from Poko with his wife and two little boys. Over half a ton of goods were packed in tight around them!

We spent a night at Isiro, and set off at six o'clock on the Wednesday morning, 27 July. Within fifty miles our troubles began. There followed 150 miles of the worst roads I had ever travelled. We struggled through deep ruts, thick mud, and pot-holes into which the whole front of the van would sink. Water channels careered crazily down every hill, cutting the road into uneven halves. We travelled, one wheel each side, weaving to and fro with the crevasses, and holding on for dear life to avoid slipping and slithering into them. The road was an endless switchback, and every hill a nightmare, every valley worse.

We travelled mainly in low gear, often in four-wheel drive, several times in low-ratio gears. We stuck twice, at a crazy 60° angle. We pushed and prayed, and ploughed through. My hands were nearly blistered, my shoulders ached. Time and again I waded through in wellington boots to measure the depth of a hole, or test the firmness of a narrow ridge.

We arrived at another Mission village, Lolwa, at 9.30 p.m., utterly exhausted, having been the first truck to make it after a terrible storm the previous night. We were held up at barriers and chatted our way through, with smiles and sweet-meats, till the soldiers laughingly waved us on.

The next morning, Thursday, on the last 50-mile lap of the long journey, we burst a tyre on the trailer! Not carrying a spare, we had to set to and repair it somehow, despite a four-inch slit right through the outer cover! We crept the last ten miles at five miles an hour, until we arrived at the large cement

83

signpost by the roadside, *Nyankunde Mission and Hope Hospital*. The words suddenly spurred us on with renewed courage. We swept up the side road for three miles' climb towards our future home, the engine roaring out our conviction of *hope* for the new adventure starting on the morrow.

Chapter 5   August 1966
You build, I teach!

Two days later I stood on the terrace outside the home where I was staying on the mountainside, and gazed out, as dawn slowly broke across the valley. The opposite hills were wrapped in low-lying mists and just the peaks reflected the pink glory of the new day. Bird-song chorused on all sides. I watched as the distant hills drew nearer, their contours rising from the dissipating mist, through the foothills to the rounded summits. The air was tangible with the fragrance of the frangipani and the stillness following heavy rain. Here and there I could see clumps of gum trees and golden acacias. Suddenly there was a vivid flash of startling blue as a weaver bird swooped by, drawing my eyes nearer across the valley. Fields of pastureland, scattered farmsteads, rounded hummock hills, the lush green following the winding river-bed, and so my eyes came to the hospital buildings below me, part hidden by bright yellow acacias and rose pink flowering shrubs. Four wards, theatre and pharmacy to my left, laboratory, X-ray and maternity to the right: beyond were the foundations of administrative and outpatient departments. Nearer, there were the pupil midwives' temporary quarters: and then just below me, and stretching up the mountainside, a wilderness of long grass and brambles, a field of some 4 to 5 acres – this was *our* school!

For a week I looked, and planned, and measured, and thought, and tried to envisage, in the place of wild elephant-grass and rough brambles, a training school for national medical auxiliaries to serve the church of the north-eastern region of Zaire. I dreamt of dispensaries opening up all over the quarter

million square miles, staffed by Zairian graduates of this school
– able, responsible, spiritual; and I saw the streams of refugees,
of hungry, naked and sick, adequately cared for by well-trained,
conscientious health officers, nurses and midwives, trained at
the Medical Centre.

I walked and stumbled in this field, measuring its slope and
realizing the difficulty of levelling and building: slithering in
its mud – thick, black, heavy alluvial soil, washed down from
the mountains, covering an impervious red-clay subsoil holding the water, damp and unsatisfactory for drainage or hygiene.
I carried the mud back home, up the hill, in inch-thick clods on
my sandals. As I gazed across the valley, imagining the immediate needs of temporary homes and class-rooms, and the future
replacements of dormitories and dining-hall, laboratories and
library, trying to see into the future, I could see only *mud*!
Acres of mud, and difficulties, and frustrations.

I had come to Nyankunde full of faith and vision and enthusiasm . . . and now, was a little bit of mud going to discourage me? No! I was sure that God had said: 'Go forward' –
and so 'go forward' we would. During the coming week I
expected students to arrive. Just how they would come was
hard to say, but we had sent out messages by modern radio and
ancient bush telegraph to invite any young men or women,
with a minimum of one year's secondary education and a desire
to serve as medical auxiliaries, to come during the first week in
August. Some who had done entrance exams probably wouldn't
turn up; others who hadn't done the exams might well turn up.
So I waited expectantly.

Meanwhile the news grew steadily more unsettled. Fighting
had broken out only 50 miles from us, between two frontier
tribes, and several were injured. One hundred miles south, a
'gang' of about one hundred armed rebels (Simbas) came down
from the mountains and attacked the population. The local
National Army lieutenant rose to the occasion and practically
wiped them out with machine-gun fire and mortars: but there
was an uneasy tension around as a result. Two wounded
National soldiers were flown to Nyankunde for surgery.

Then we heard that, to the north, another missionary and his
wife had had their new 6-ton diesel lorry commandeered.

Katangese and mercenary troops appeared to be pouring into Kisangani from all sides, and whites were said to have been evacuated. Some even added that all 'Simbas' in prison had been liberated and given arms. Greeks added to the gloom by telling us that Isiro had been stripped bare and all vehicles commandeered by the mercenaries. They said that all whites had fled the area, several over the border into the Central African Republic.

Added to this sort of news, we had our own 'extras' in the way of fairly violent earth-tremors, almost daily. Nyankunde had been considerably shaken in March 1966 by the earthquake that hit the Ruwenzori mountain range, and these rumblings now shook our hills fairly constantly.

Despite the happenings around us, the medical team went ahead and held their first official meeting of the 'Board of Directors'. It lasted from 11.0 a.m. to 9.0 p.m.! We drew up statutes for the new inter-mission medical project, got everything decently translated into correct French and typed up in five copies. Now we really felt officially 'launched'!

I filled in time while awaiting the arrival of students by visiting the local chieftain to pay my respects, and to ask permission to cut poles in his afforestation area, at 3p for a 10-foot pole. We needed some 1,500 such poles for the plan I had made out for our initial building programme. I also managed a trip to our local township of Bunia, some 30 miles to the north-east, to lay in stores for the school kitchen. It was quite exciting thinking and ordering in large quantities, such as half a ton of rice, ten sacks of flour and ten of sugar, ten cartons of soap at a hundred pieces each, forty-gallon drums of petrol, paraffin and palm oil: besides looking at bales of cloth and blankets, dozens of buckets, bowls, lanterns, mugs and plates, huge cartons of matches – there seemed no end to the list.

And then *they* came! There were twenty-two students in the first batch. I can still picture them as they arrived. Manassé, tall, debonair, light-skinned, wearing sun-glasses and looking down from some lofty height of self-importance – he managed to make me feel very small! Jack, short and thick-set, very dark-skinned, not bright judging by his entrance paper, but with an air of knowing all the answers which I found a little intimidating – accompanied by a quiet, inoffensive little wife and four rowdy children. Peter – oh, dear me! – from the first, Peter and I clashed. I remember one day in class: two of us staff were struggling to keep three classes going, and we were teaching in shifts, from 6.30 a.m. till 8.30 p.m. every day. It was necessary to make some slight adjustment in their time-tables to allow Miss Fuchsloch to fit in the necessary hours of practical supervision in the wards. The change was written up on the blackboard, and Peter stood and drawled, in his near-perfect French, with a superb disdain for the usual student/ staff relationship: 'Has the Government approved this change?' The class held their breath, never quite sure whose side to take. I held my breath and counted ten – and then quietly replied that the Government had *suggested* the change. A gasp – and then the class clapped, and the bubble was pricked for that round – but there were many such rounds in the ensuing two years.

I remember most clearly those who gave most challenge, but there were others: quiet, gracious Joel, who had been with me at Nebobongo before the Rebellion and stood by me fear-lessly when I was nearly killed – back now to finish his courses, with his unobtrusive young wife; Joseph and Canisius, Ruandese refugees, taller than the Zairians, a little aloof per-haps, or else only shy and reserved, good-looking young men, hard workers, always courteous and helpful; Job, dull and heavy – he had not passed the entrance exam and we never quite knew how he got in, except that he came with the crowd from the south with a 'good story' – but he never quite rang true to me; Seth, small and wiry, like a house sparrow, bright as a button in appearance and speech, but completely the reverse where academic achievement was concerned! How he ever passed the entrance exam remains a mystery, unless he had been helped by Jack. He became known to everyone by his invariable response to each and every request throughout his three years with us: 'No problem, no problem' – and then, equally invariably, a howler would follow.

They had arrived in groups of four and five, each group from different directions. Some were chatting nonchalantly, self-possessed: they felt they knew the ropes and were just coming to continue their ordinary way of life, but in our set-up: they knew the medical director, Dr Becker, and were prepared to show other newcomers what to do. Others were shy, withdrawn into themselves, very fearful of this new start in their lives. Yet others, like Peter, were proud and rather disdainful – they had already completed three years of secondary school and considered themselves a cut above the rest, a little unsure whether we were worthy of the honour of their presence.

Nevertheless all were tired, dirty and hungry. The fortunate few had been brought the hundred miles down the escarpment by car, Manassé among them: the less fortunate had spent five days hitch-hiking in transport lorries over 300 miles of wild jungle country, often helping to push the heavily-laden vehicles through seas of mud, or even to unload and later re-load their transport truck in deluging rain, for a spring to be repaired. A few local students, such as Joel, had cycled or walked across the valley, carrying their precious bundles of all they possessed tied up in bright-coloured cloths, or packed in rough soap boxes. All were expectant, wondering, and a little dazed after two years of suffering to be given this chance to continue their schooling.

Two years ago, some of these were in our Nebobongo nursing aids' school; others were in different primary and secondary schools throughout the region; ordinary, teenage students, happy, free ... they didn't have much in the way of clothes, or housing, or personal possessions, but that didn't count much. They studied when they felt like it, and played when they didn't! Football was more important than textbooks: yet at the end of each year, like students all the world over, they suddenly became stuck to their books, the football field deserted: and then, all smiling, they passed their final exams with flying colours and looking as though they thought they deserved it!

And then the holocaust of the civil war, the Simba Rebellion, had swept across their horizon, absorbing everything before it. They were the lucky ones, still alive – many, many of their classmates were gone, killed, murdered, liquidated. They had seen whole class-rooms of fourteen-year-olds rounded up, herded into waiting lorries, driven off to the 'front' – singing, shouting slogans, their morale boosted by liquor and drugs, and the pledge of the power of witchcraft to bring them back victorious. Hardly any had returned. And these others, after two years of hide-and-seek in the dense forest, avoiding involvement in the tragedy of war, had survived and were seeking to pick up the threads again.

Slowly they gathered in the driveway behind Dr Becker's house. I took their names and welcomed them, sitting at a camp table on a wooden chair in the open yard. In front of us was *our* field, 5 acres of steeply-sloping land in the bowl of the hills, shoulder-high with rough grass and thornbush, and huge clumps of elephant-grass towering above. Their eyes strayed across the valley, wondering where the school was, where the dormitories, as I and John Mangadima, once again my assistant director, gave out blankets, plates, mugs and spoons, lamps and bowls, matches and soap.

Manassé strolled forward from the group. 'Where is the school, Doctor?'

With as cool a wave of the arm as I could manage, indicating the field and rising mountain-slopes, 'Over there,' I replied.

Their eyes slowly turned and followed my pointing hand.

'And the dormitories?' Manassé continued, refusing to show any reaction.

'Also there,' I replied, my eyes now challenging his for further comments. It began to sink in – there *was* no school, no dormitories. Yet . . . hadn't I invited them to come? For the moment I left the subject, and turned to the immediate needs of sleeping accommodation for that first night.

The local headmaster was lending us two primary-school class-rooms during the summer holidays; several church elders had offered to house one or two students; some of the missionaries managed to squeeze in one or two in their already overflowing homes. As we called each name and assigned them to a home or room or dormitory, we were conscious of mutterings and murmurings, and I seriously wondered if we were going to be able to win them round. These young men, mostly seventeen to twenty years old, all secondary-schoolboys, representing nine different tribes, from six different church areas and backgrounds, presented us with a tremendous challenge. Could we win their confidence? And would they trust us to direct them during the coming crucial years? Not only were they young men at the cross-roads of their individual lives, but they were young citizens at the cross-roads of emerging African nationalism. The problems seemed to loom higher than the elephant-grass. These proud young men, full of their own importance at having secondary-school education, with all the determination to assert their independence, would they agree to weed, and clear, and cut, and build?

Later that afternoon they drifted back, and we surveyed the valley together. We pushed our way through the tangled undergrowth, measuring out ten-yard plots. Then we scrambled up another steep rise through a forest of elephant-grass and came out on a small level platform, and, laughing and breathless, looked back down the valley. 'That is our school,' I said, with a sweep of the hand across the waving green maze. Students eyed me quizzically, some almost hostilely. Could I be serious? Again they looked at the waste below us, and ourselves heavy with thick black mud, and our clothes full of thorns and burrs. And I appealed to them openly.

'You build, I teach.'

Are you willing to get your shirts off, take up the tools, and turn that valley into a school village by sheer, dogged, hard labour? Will you clear and dig and weed the ground? Will you go out into the afforestation areas, 6 to 10 miles away, and fell trees, hauling them back on your bare shoulders? Will you build and roof and thatch? Will you stick at it till we have a school village to house us all and all the families of our married students? *Then* I will teach you – my word, I may not know much French, I may know even less about politics and economics, but I can teach, and those of you who want to learn to be dressers, orderlies, nurses, health officers, medical auxiliaries, I'll teach you all I've got!

A stunned silence met me, as the reality of the proposition sank into their minds. So I really was serious. This was no joke, no white man's sense of humour. I actually meant it: 'You build, I teach.' It was fantastic. It just couldn't be real. Some closed their eyes and shook their heads, as though to shake off an unpleasant nightmare.

'We'll meet tomorrow at 6.30 a.m. in the courtyard for your decision,' I said jovially, inwardly quaking with doubts lest they would not respond. So we made our several ways down the hillside to our homes in search of an evening meal.

There was a special welcome service arranged in the church that evening, led by church elders and medical staff, Zairians and foreigners. The students all came, possibly as they had nowhere else to go. The theme was 'workers together with God'. Slowly, as different ones spoke and through the singing of the hymns, I felt some of the students begin to thaw towards us, accepting the challenge. Others, however, remained withdrawn, their eyes wary and suspicious, if not actually hostile.

Next morning dawned misty with drizzling rain. I went out to the courtyard and rigged up a couple of planks on some broken cement-blocks that I rolled into position. I put out my chair and camp table, and sat down to wait for the students. I began reading my Bible, a short morning portion. They did not come, and my reading continued to the end of the chapter. Still they didn't come, and I continued to the end of the book. I was wet and chilled, and very nearly discouraged. So much lay in the balance.

During the previous week many of the legal representatives and senior men, African and European, of the six participating mission/churches had met to form an administrative council. During the meetings I had proposed that the students themselves should build their own temporary homes in the school village. If we started at once, building through August and September, I reckoned we could start classes in October 1966.

My proposal had met with incredulity and open laughter!

All the available finance at the Centre was already allocated for wards, outpatient departments, homes for the missionary staff, drug supplies, medical and surgical equipment. The school would have ended the list. We should have to wait till the fall of 1967 to get started. But I was impatient. My own particular 'bee in the bonnet' had always been that 'no white man is justified in working in Black Africa unless he/she is teaching'. I could see no ultimate justification for the Medical

Centre, except for the college. There had to be a Centre as the college could not function without the hospital and all its ancillary departments; but equally, there must be the college to give the Centre credence.

But could I really build the school with nothing? The other council members were justifiably sceptical. It must have sounded a wild-cat scheme. Strangely enough, no-one actually asked me how much *money* I had available or how I would feed the students during the three months of building or how I would procure the necessary supplies for the first term. No, the one burning question had been: 'Do you honestly believe that you, a foreigner, and a woman into the bargain, can persuade secondary-schoolboys, nineteen/twenty-year-old youths, with a consciousness of their own dignity as the "white collar" workers of the future, to build?' No-one asked me what I knew of building myself, nor who would measure out the land, plan the over-all development, collect the materials, construct the homes. No, they had just asked: 'Can you make *students* do it, willingly?'

And I had staked my reputation on it.

At 8.45 a.m. that first morning they arrived, and I had won!

I tried to pretend that I hadn't noticed they were over two hours late. I tried to ignore the fact that I was wet through with waiting in the drizzle. I tried to appear as though there was no question hanging in the air. We sang a hymn; I gave my prepared Bible study; then I started assigning work. The students let out their breath. I don't know where they had met, who was their leader, what led them in the end to agree with my proposal; but it was obvious that they had agreed, even though they said nothing.

In a businesslike way we divided ourselves into three groups. Each group had a set of tools and appointed a group leader. One group of nine had axes to go to the nearest afforestation area and fell trees; the next had hoes to clear a dormitory site. The third had knife-like scythes to mow down the jungle of tall grass to the south of the dormitories, where we would start a football field and, beyond, food-gardens. Granted there was not much enthusiasm, and it was soon apparent that some had never handled an axe before. They certainly were an ignorant bunch where building was concerned. But suddenly someone said: 'O.K. You win – we build and you teach!' and everyone started laughing at the sheer impossibility of the suggestion.

The ice was thawed, the tension gone, and I began teaching in earnest how to handle tools. We drew up the plans together, we paced out the land together, we marked off the plots, and I offered a bonus prize to the first group to complete their assignment. Two groups of nine youths each, to the two dormitories, each with a 6-yard deep toilet-pit: and ultimately five groups of three married men each, to do three small homes, each with cookhouse and toilet. They even managed to become excited. But in no time their unaccustomed hands were raw and sore, and it wasn't always easy to keep them at it from 6.30 a.m. through to 5.30 p.m. each day.

I went out with the first crew of tree-fellers, walking the three miles across the rough hillside to the nearest afforestation area. We worked all day in twos, an axe between each pair, felling blue gums (eucalyptus) anything from 6 to 18 inches in diameter, and some 25 feet high. As they fell crashing to the ground, the second of each pair lopped off all side branches, clearing these of leaves and smaller branches, and stacking them for roofing framework. The first day, in our enthusiasm and ignorance, we overdid it, and as dusk quickly fell we were suddenly all of us just too dog-tired to make the journey home. We lay out there on the mountainside between the poles we had cut, and slept soundly. By next morning I was so stiff and sore that it was hard to believe we would ever achieve our target. We struggled home in the early morning dawn for breakfast – and were inwardly furious to find that no-one had missed us, let alone considered sending out a search party for us!

We made the most of every encouragement: the first poles erected called for 20 gallons of sweetened tea! The first roof on (it was Jack's house – they fêted him, but there was a gnawing corner of suspicion in my heart that he hadn't really acted honourably. The other homes in his group were far behind, and he was obviously working as a lone wolf and not as a member

94

of a team, often a danger sign) demanded an afternoon off for a football match!

We pulled together, and slowly the students began to realize that we *could* do it. Neat rows of houses began to appear; each day toilet-pits went down a few more hard-earned inches, and we felt ourselves approaching our target-date for completion. It was the driest wet-season on record, or we could never have got that far. Others willingly helped us, hauling in lumber at all hours, or preparing meals for us. This involved more problems, as students from the north had never eaten the local manioc porridge and southerners could not stomach the palm oil; several said they could not digest corn flour, or beans, or other items of staple diet. But again, we learnt together.

The political news those days – or rather, the lack of news – was disturbing and distressing. The mercenary and Katangese units in the National Army were in mutinous revolt against Colonel Mobutu, the Head of State. Kisangani was cut off from us, and four prospective students from that area still had not arrived. Isiro was likewise cut off, and the eleven prospective students from the old Nebobongo school, coming directly into their third year of studies, still had not come. Mail arrived only intermittently, and told us of the evacuation of missionaries and Europeans from both these towns. A general sense of tension underlay everything, and one felt that at any moment a spark could ignite a new conflagration.

Then sickness attacked us, to add to our difficulties. Several students went down with severe bouts of malaria; then bacillary dysentery put nine boys on their beds for several days; then two developed typhoid fever. We were well into September, and really only half-way through our project. I wanted to provide decent eating and sleeping accommodation before starting classes. But it was clear to me that we would need three months to create a habitable village, especially as work now slowed down considerably for ten days. Small problems began to loom large. Grumbling started over the food rations, the housing conditions, the long hours I drove the students to keep them at the building. We had to evacuate the primary-school buildings at the start of their new term, before our own first dormitory was ready. Tribal differences reared their head and became focused in the missing group from Nebobongo. The former students were all WaBudus by tribe, as was John Mangadima, my assistant director.

When it was obvious that classes would not start on 1 October and I proposed to postpone the official school opening till 31 October, feeling was running dangerously high. Someone muttered: 'She's holding out for her WaBudu students to arrive.'

So I temporized: 'O.K., let's aim at 15 October – see if we can finish in ten weeks from starting.'

Then we had a fortnight of torrential rains. Our fields became a quagmire. Roads were impassable for hauling poles. Grass, urgently needed for thatching, was beaten down and damaged. Morning after morning we woke to drenching mists shrouding the hills and soaking the valley, only to be displaced by heavy banks of dark, scudding clouds with more rain and yet more rain. It needed so much courage to believe we would ever finish!

Meanwhile, in between measuring and checking, weighing and building, and a multitude of other jobs to help the project forward, there was also a mountain of office-work to be done. Each student needed a personal file prepared, with past and present details of educational attainments, plus family history, medical records, and a word on his spiritual state. Accounts had to be kept, for all the building material, transport costs, kitchen utensils, food, soap, paraffin and firewood, and all the essential equipment for starting a new secondary school. Lectures had to be prepared, time-tables arranged, and a hundred and one other responsibilities seen to, often between eight and eleven o'clock at night.

As the work neared the end, the problems seemed to intensify and multiply. Manassé walked off one day, over his strong-willed refusal to eat beans. The group of students working on the southern dormitory became sullen, as their building had to be taken down and re-done due to carelessness. Their determination to finish first had allowed slackness in accuracy, and poles were not properly measured, so that the roof-supporting poles were not absolutely horizontal. Had we allowed this building to continue, the roof-thatching would not have stood up to the heavy tropical storms for the length of time we planned, so those responsible were told to pull it down, and they didn't like it. Within a few days the Mission's 5-ton lorry and the Medical Centre's tractor, both heavily laden with roof-truss poles, twine and grass, were bogged down four miles away in thick mud.

By the end of that week, however, Manassé returned – with a letter from an elderly lady missionary who had brought him up in a church orphanage, to say that he honestly could not eat beans, and we agreed to supplement his diet with animal protein. The southern dormitory group rallied and made a tremendous effort, working late into the evenings, to catch up with their northerly neighbours – and we helped them all Saturday afternoon (while the others played football) to fasten the roof-timbers in place. Our Land Rover went out and succeeded in towing the tractor up the hill, and eventually helped to deliver all the lumber we needed to complete the frameworks to our village buildings.

At the same time as all this, other activities were pushing forward. We cleared paths up the mountainside and staked out twenty-eight plots for food-gardens. We completed clearing a full-sized football field and attempted to level it a bit. We employed a local village tailor to get going on making shirts and shorts and aprons for the nursing students. Considerable time was spent three times a week at local markets bargaining for our food needs. With no difficulty at all I found sixteen hours a day full of activity and sufficiently hard work to ensure eight hours' solid sleep by night – and no time left for preparing lectures.

After almost continuous rain for seventeen days the sun returned, and work went forward again at a pace. The students were finding it easier now to do ten hours' hard work, without blisters or grumbles. But the opening date had been put back once more to 30 October and I could sense annoyance and frustration in many of them. So I wasn't altogether taken by surprise at their next move, even if hurt by their lack of trust and seeming unreasonableness.

A representation of each of the three proposed classes for the coming year, with John Mangadima as spokesman, went to see Dr Becker, the medical director of the Centre, with four main questions, which he sought to answer both fairly and clearly.

'Who is finally in charge of the school?' And one sensed the underlying question: 'Can Dr Roseveare expel a student, or have we a higher court of appeal?'

Dr Becker replied: 'Dr Roseveare has been appointed school director by the unanimous vote of the Administrative Council, African and foreign leaders of the participating churches and missions,' and we stored away the knowledge that a disciplinary committee would have to be created as a satisfactory court of appeal.

'Why has the date of commencement of lectures been several times put off?' If the first question had raised an optimistic hope of intelligence, the second reversed this, as the answer seemed so obvious: 'The change of the date of commencement is due to the unsettled condition of your own country and through no fault of the missionary,' not even mentioning that we had been quite unprepared earlier, with no homes, no books, no lectures.

'Why can we not start school till the northern students arrive?' They were speaking of those from the Nebobongo area, delayed by the mutiny in the army causing transport chaos in their area. These students were mainly for second- and third-year classes, having begun their studies before the Rebellion. All were from the Nebobongo church area and mostly of the WaBudu tribe; and the question really meant, 'Is favouritism going to be shown to the WaBudu students, at the expense of the others?'

Amongst those expected from Nebobongo was the church elder appointed to be bursar/chaplain to our new school, Basuana, who had been with me during the previous twelve years. Dr Becker replied calmly: 'Obviously Dr Roseveare needs the school administrator to relieve her of many of her multitudinous duties if she is to be free to teach you in the class-room.'

Finally, 'Who has arranged the programme?' they asked, almost belligerently. In other words, was the whole plan merely a whim of mine, a fantasy, a hair-brained scheme, or could they be assured of receiving Government recognition at the end?

Now I myself longed for real satisfaction on this point! But the Government, who had given many verbal promises, had sent no letter, no statement, no signature. They just were not prepared to commit themselves. It was all a gigantic gamble – yet I felt a spiritual assurance that God was saying 'Go ahead'. But could one build a school on that? Could one ask intelligent youths to risk their future on that? To put in four years of studies, paying school fees, for a mythical diploma and therefore a precarious salary at the end?

'Dr Roseveare spent three weeks, at her own expense, on your behalf in Kinshasa searching out and obtaining the official Government programme, and pledges of full recognition.'

They were partly satisfied, though still suspicious. One could not blame their suspicions. I sensed the struggle of the newly-independent against the feared 'neo-colonialist', and yet their hunger for the education I could give them. It wasn't going to be easy for them or for me.

At last, however, the initial building programme was practically completed. Water-piping brought fresh drinking-water to the village from the mountains. A 48-foot flagpole was cut, cleaned and erected in the centre of the compound. Rubbish was cleared away; final touches put to finished buildings – 'hair-cuts', as we called it, given to the thatches; shirts and shorts were issued to the thirty two male students, and blue-and-white striped dresses to the three girls; household equipment was provided for each of the eighteen married students. Some of their wives and children began to arrive.

Yet there was still no sign of the northern students, or of Basuana who would carry all the administrative load of the village, and so release me for the duties of the class-room. Could I go forward without him? Yet rising tensions among a few of the strong-minded students made us feel it was imperative to get going on 'Phase two'.

Chapter 6 October 1966
So we were launched

On Saturday 29 October, three months after we had started building the school village, we dedicated the college with a moving flag-raising ceremony, and launched out into the job of teaching.

Thirty-six students had arrived by then, and some two-thirds of the initial temporary-building programme had been completed. During the last week of October there was a sudden rush of final tidying – weeding, digging, sweeping, planting bright red canna lilies – to have the central courtyard cleared and each house standing in its own neat area. Fifteen missionaries and many Zairian colleagues had gathered on the newly-cut road to the north of the village for the simple ceremony. The thirty-six young men in smart airforce-blue shirts with school pocket-badges, and olive-green shorts, and our first three girl students in blue-and-white pin-striped dresses, marched into the compound forming a large semicircle around the flagpole.

We sang; Dr Becker and others prayed; John Mangadima unfurled our new flag; Jack Sibaminya blew heartily on an ancient trumpet. All came smartly to attention for the National Anthem as the flag rose slowly to the top of the mast, uncurled and waved out bravely against a clear blue sky.

Suddenly the moment passed, solemnity disappeared, and dignified students turned into ardent footballers. Blue shirts and hymnbooks were speedily exchanged for white T-shirts and a ball, and 'marrieds' played 'singles'.

'Well, how do you feel now?' one senior missionary jocularly quizzed me over a cup of tea. 'Not bad, eh? You made it, despite all we prophesied!'

I hesitated, and sensed a sudden wave of fear: I was scared. There had been difficult, even tense, moments during the past three months – as one might expect amongst any group of thirty-six senior teenagers. Yet I felt suddenly sick with apprehension. Could we carry out what we had set our hands to? The whole scheme seemed so futile, really, looked at worldly-wise. Here was I, intensely proud of my developing new village, but in the cool light of reason I knew that it resembled a corner of the slums, over-crowded, extremely poor, muddy, and inevitably underfed. Why had I done it? My whole being had always longed to give the Africans as good as the Europeans had. We called our village 'temporary', but it had cost a cool £1,000 already, and finance was running out.

Could I really run the school and the administration? What if Basuana did not come? Was my own knowledge any longer up to today's required standard of teaching? The difference between American and British medical methods appeared to be considerable. Was I sufficiently adaptable to be willing to teach in theory as the Americans would be doing in practice? I suddenly felt very small and very weary. Was I young enough to carry the load any longer, and the long strenuous hours which would undoubtedly be involved?

'Helen,' chided a colleague, 'a penny for your thoughts!'

'Not worth it!' I exclaimed with a grin, and came back to earth and the job of pouring out cups of tea.

So we were launched.

I remember that first Sunday, marching three abreast the half mile from school to church, all dressed alike with maroon trousers or skirts and white shirts – startling, to put it mildly! Certainly eye-catching, and I dared not turn my head to catch the varying expressions as we passed an admiring crowd. Some were curious, some sceptical, some amused no doubt: and yet probably all were hopeful that this hailed a new start. Dr Becker preached that morning, and John Mangadima gave a short word of personal testimony. It was a good service, and the student body seemed attentive and interested.

Liliane Fuchsloch had arrived back from furlough in Switzerland, in time for the opening ceremony. She was to become deeply involved in the teaching programme of the college, practical and theoretical. We had walked all over the new school compound, discussing all the plans and proposals. We had visited the new hospital and dispensary sites, and the old dispensary buildings. These, we felt, could be converted without too much difficulty into class-rooms, to serve until our own new buildings were ready. We spent hours discussing courses and time-tables.

Liliane had already completed two terms of service at Nyankunde and in the immediate vicinity. She had served the local community as nurse and midwife, and had helped on the staff of the nursing aids' school which had previously been at Nyankunde, from 1955 to 1960. She knew something of the pressures of time-tables involving theory and practical classes, lectures and supervision, with insufficient staff. She was French-speaking by birth, and knew something of the pain of listening to British and Americans hashing up her language in the wards. Could she stand it also in the class-rooms? The radical changes that I and others were so glibly suggesting were to a work dear to her heart, that she had helped to build up and establish. How would she take it all?

'I think it is magnificent!' she exclaimed enthusiastically, as we finally got back to my room and a cup of coffee. From then on we worked closely together, and found we were on each other's wave-length!

We prayed over each decision and sought God's mind together on each problem facing us. We were both conscious that the coming year might prove decisive in the history of Zaire. No-one knew how long we had in which to offer any help in re-establishing educational and medical services. Would the whole economic structure crumble? Would the malcontents start a counter-revolution? Would the ultra-nationalists insist on the withdrawal of all foreigners before we could hand over properly?

It was no good theorizing. I could be neither philosophical nor political. There was a job to be done and we set about doing it. After that first Sunday of dedication, we had two days for final preparations before classes were to start on the Wednesday. We cleared an old store-room that the church was lending us as a class-room. We arranged shelves, desks and forms, made by a local carpenter. We found two tables and chairs. We 'blacked' some boards, sorted exercise and textbooks, pencils and blackboard chalk, all brought out from England nine months before. The carpenter mended two broken window-frames and made fixtures for our charts and models. Two missionaries installed electricity for us, with a line from the generator which served the local printing press. Liliane and I completed what preparation we could give to the time-tables, drew up a simple set of rules for the school, created a committee from local national church members and medical staff, and planned staff meetings for routine school direction.

So the stage was set and our training college launched. On the Wednesday at 6.30 a.m. the students assembled, all in their new nurses' uniforms, all expectant and curious, some probably a little fearful. Afer an opening hymn of praise I spoke briefly on our college motto: 'Unto Him, without limits' taken from the Campaigner youth movement, of which most of our senior students were keen members. We tried to set out clearly and deliberately (albeit in hesitant French) the aims and ideals of the college. It was being formed as part of the local church to train them, not only as medical auxiliaries, but also as Christian evangelists. Our standards and rules were unashamedly based on the Bible. In our opinion, as staff, whole-hearted commitment by each individual to the keeping of God's first and great commandment: 'The Lord our God, the Lord is one; and you shall love the Lord your God with all your heart, and with all your soul, and with all your mind, and with all your strength,' would knit us together as a family, and create from the outset the right sort of atmosphere that the college hoped for.

As I was writing my diary at the end of that first week, jotting down a few of the manifold happenings and listing the jobs that must have priority in the coming week, there was a great longing in my heart for the arrival of our eleven students from the north with Basuana Bernard, our college bursar. These senior students needed to get into classes at once with no further loss of time if they were to complete their courses in the year. Basuana was urgently needed to take over the oversight of the kitchens, the tailors, the new building programme and a hundred and one other jobs that I was still having to do between and after classes.

Suddenly my thoughts and day-dreaming were shattered.

'They've come!'

The courtyard was full of crazy noise – laughing, singing and crying. We helped them down from the lorry, thick with mud, weary from sixty hours on the road, many painfully thin from two years of under-nourishment, several sick and feverish. Many of the younger children were fretful, sore from the bruising treatment of the truck over the atrocious roads, through days of deluging rain. Basuana, eleven students, plus the six wives, twelve children and all their goods were eventually disgorged into the drive, to a tumultuous welcome.

There was Basuana, solid and tough at forty, utterly reliable and loyal, my right-hand man through our ten years together at Nebobongo, up to and during the Rebellion. He had been school chaplain and administrator as well as maintenance man and my own close friend. His wife Andugui and five of their nine children were with him. He just stepped straight into my shoes, and carried all the burdens of building, feeding and direction with a quiet, unruffled efficiency.

On the second morning after their arrival, at breakfast-time, he came to me with a list in his hand.

'Doctor, I've just checked the tool-shed. Three axes, five hoes and two machetes are missing. May I have permission to put a padlock on the door and keep an inventory?'

I swallowed my desire to apologize for my inefficiency and told him to go ahead, fine by me!

At the end of that week he came again with another list.

'Doctor, we really need to employ a second cook for the school kitchens, and a couple of gardeners for the school food-gardens. I've interviewed several people, and suggest we take on the following for a month's trial.'

Again I gulped and grinned. It was good to have him back, and this sounded like old times!

'Go ahead, boss. Fine by me.'

All I was asked to do was to sign their contract in their work-books and to pay them at the end of the month!

On the following Thursday three students arrived from the 'big city', as we called Kisangani, the capital of our north-eastern region. They came into class at 8.15 p.m., just as we were about to start evening prayers. They were given a tremendous welcome by everyone, escorted back to the village where they were taken to the dormitories, given a bed each with mattress and blankets, and then served a hot meal. How different from our arrival three months earlier, when not a single building was yet erected, and no hot meal available!

But the next morning two of the three were waiting for me when I returned from school at eleven o'clock. They were full of complaints.

'Don't you realize that we have already done two years' secondary school? Why should we start again in first-year studies?' grumbled the lads, revealing their ignorance by their inability to comprehend that any new course of studies must start at its own first year.

'Don't you understand that we are *secondary* schoolboys, and therefore should not be asked to *build*? And anyway, if we should build, you would certainly be obliged to pay us full wages.'

I was just weighing up how to tackle their attitude when they continued belligerently: 'and the food! We have been accustomed to . . .', but I found that I had switched off, so to speak. This was what we had been given to expect from any coming from the 'big city', in sharp contrast to the gratitude of the forest-born students.

I allowed them to continue in their own strain, asking a question here and there, or expressing a doubt in the midst of their reasoning, for about an hour, and then felt I had had enough.

'Are you, or are you not, called by God to be medical auxiliaries? We are at present the only college in this vast region accepting students for any of the three possible option courses. If you are called to this service, you'd be well to accept what we offer and settle down. If not, it is well that you leave before I enter your names on the register.'

I suggested that they should leave me then, and come back at 2.30 p.m. when my assistant director would be with me. John and I sent for them at three o'clock only to learn that they had already left.

On Sunday 6 November I went the 30 miles to our nearest town of Bunia, after morning service, to meet the midday plane. We were eagerly expecting Jill Thompstone, an English nurse/midwife with teaching qualifications, who was coming to work at the Medical Centre on the college staff. However, there was no-one on the plane that I knew, not an uncommon experience where plane services were concerned!

Most days my waking hours, from 5.0 a.m. with coffee till nearly midnight, were packed tight with activity. School hours were from 6.30 a.m. morning prayers to nine o'clock evening prayers just before the generators were turned off for the night. We managed twelve lecture-periods between the three different classes, with meal breaks and school staff meetings sandwiched in between. Then home to light pressure-lanterns, and to start marking books and preparing tomorrow's lectures. Through the first four years this daily preparation continued, always for tomorrow's lectures. We never seemed to be able to get ahead of ourselves. The subjects had to be decided on, read up, thought over, simplified, written out, translated into French, typed on stencils and run through the duplicator, the latter process sometimes being at about one o'clock in the morning.

At first the French was a tremendous strain for me. Until the Rebellion I had used French only sparingly, talking mainly in Swahili, the trade language. Now French was obligatory for all secondary school and higher education. I was never quite sure how much of what I said the students followed, nor how extensive was their limited vocabulary. Each Saturday we gave simple test papers, often on the multiple-choice question system, in each subject, on the one week's work, just to encourage them to study regularly throughout the year. These began to reveal how much (or how little) they understood. One of the best howlers during the first month was an answer to a geography question in the general knowledge paper, 'Describe the structure of the earth.' One student wrote: 'A nucleus of molten metals, surrounded by a sort of cement-paste to hold people on, so they won't fall off.' An attempt, perhaps, to explain magnetic force?

At last, on Saturday 19 November, Jill Thompstone arrived! We were thrilled to welcome her. Once the students heard her near-perfect French, they gave her an even warmer welcome than the staff had done! When Liliane and I prepared the year's time-tables, we had prepared one for Jill along with ours. Jill had been preparing for her life's work as a sister-tutor in Zaire for a considerable time, as she had been delayed two years by the events of the Rebellion. Now that she had arrived, she was as excited as we were to get launched.

Then, ten days after her arrival, one Monday morning, Dr Becker sent for us. He reminded us of the urgent, almost desperate need of the hospital for trained nursing help. In other words: 'Couldn't you and Liliane carry the teaching programme for this first term, or even the whole first year, without Jill's help, Helen?'

Dr Becker's eyes seemed to bore into me, and yet held an urgent sense of appeal. Just for a brief moment I reeled as under a physical blow. We had so counted on Jill's aid to cut the heavy hours of teaching and preparation: but I could see clearly the force of all the arguments he began to assemble. Without an efficiently-run hospital, our students could not receive the necessary training. Jill herself would obviously benefit by working, for a time at least, in the hospital under our local tropical conditions, before trying to teach the students techniques suitable for African nursing practice.

I glanced quickly at Jill, and sensed the fight in her heart. She was longing to get into the teaching for which she was specially trained, and to which she had been looking forward for so long. Yet she was willing to fit in where she was most needed. I caught her eye, and we smiled as we understood so exactly what was going through each other's mind. Together we agreed to Dr Becker's proposal. That very afternoon Jill went to take over responsibility as theatre sister, continuing to give her mornings to language study and evenings to helping prepare lectures.

Another job Jill offered to take on immediately was to sort

out the college accounts! I had tried almost in vain to balance these, between all the other activities. I never had been much good at this, back in my Nebobongo days, and obviously I had not improved at the exercise over the years. The vastness of the figures now involved, compared to those old days, staggered me. In the first four months we had gone through over £1,000 in freewill offerings and personal gifts from friends at home.

'Phew! If it has taken that much just to launch us, whatever is it going to take to keep us afloat?'

Somewhat daunted, I had fought on at the books, to get them ready to hand over to Jill in the New Year. Looking back and reviewing the achievement of those first four months, I was not only thinking of the £1,000 finance, but also of all the nervous effort, as well as physical, that had gone into each aspect of the initial building programme and launching. Could we really achieve what we were aiming at, in the eight years that I had specified at Kinshasa in May? The mountain of difficulties seemed almost insurmountable – physical, material, financial, medical and spiritual.

The next day a letter came out of the blue, to encourage us. It was from the American consul in Kinshasa, proposing to give the college some financial help from their American A.I.D. (self-help) programme, on certain conditions. We, the college authorities, must guarantee the balance of the finance needed to complete the building programme; it must be completed in 'reasonable time'; and we must employ local voluntary labour, including the students. It was an encouragement, certainly, but also a challenge. Could we accept the conditions?

In Friday school, during the daily hour given to general science and applied mathematics, I took the students into our confidence and explained what might be involved by the proposed conditions. Together we drew up scale-plans of the proposed new college complex, class-rooms, offices and laboratory block, dining-hall, kitchen and stores block, dormitories and living quarters, and finally sports facilities and grounds. We prepared a budget, including the hiring of a contractor, ordering materials, paying workmen and transport. I explained the need to submit progress reports to all those financing the project. The students easily became more excited than I was, as they conveniently could not see all the thousands of snags and difficulties that might crop up.

As they worked on their plans, I was busily calculating how many tons of cement we would need, how many thousands of bricks, sheets of asbestos roofing, cubic metres of timber, panes of glass. I was reckoning out the cost of masons and assistants at the present scale of salaries, how many weeks of labour would be involved, and how many miles of transport. Multiplying, adding, subtracting. I decided not to contract out to anyone but to 'do-it-yourself'. Eventually I came up with a tentative figure of costs per square metre of surface area. Then reckoning on inevitable rises in costs of materials and wages, the figure began to look astronomical, in the realm of £25,000 for the total project. Over a five-year period, that would be £5,000 annually, and this to be divided between the five main mission/churches participating in the Centre. I began to get excited too, as I realized that it *could* be done.

I tried to explain to the students that the 20,000 hours of free labour that they had already contributed while building the temporary village could be counted in balance to this new permanent project, even though this would have to be done by skilled paid labour. That they found harder to understand, but decided to take my word for it, when they discovered that this meant they were not being asked to contribute more hours of labour!

Had I known then that costs of material would quadruple and salaries treble before the project was through; that months would pass with no cement or other vital commodity available; weeks possibly with no-one available for a particular job needing specialist skills; that Zaire currency, and later both the dollar and sterling, would lose their value – I might not have been quite so sanguine in signing my name to the American A.I.D. proposal. Perhaps it is just as well in this life that we do not know too much about tomorrow while we still have today with us. Suffice it to say that, six years after signing that contract and accepting an initial gift of £2,000, the programme was almost completed in every detail. But we faced formidable and unforeseen problems along the way.

Chapter 7   1966-1967

Extra-curricular activities

Sundays began to take on a particular pattern. The students had been going out preaching each week with a local church elder in another missionary's vehicle. One Sunday I was woken at 6.20 a.m. to be told that the chauffeur who drove the students to the surrounding villages was ill: could I please drive them? Momentarily displeased at being woken so early on a Sunday, after working till after midnight every day the previous week, I checked a hasty comment and got dressed. After a quick cup of coffee I drove down the hill in the Land Rover to collect some eight or ten students, and then thought of Jill. I ran across to her room and tapped on the window.

'Jill, we're going out preaching in the villages up the Irumu road. Would you like to come with us?' – and in five minutes she was there!

It was a perfectly lovely day, clear, with a low heat-haze over the hills and a cloudless pale blue sky. Jill and I chatted in English as we went, mainly of the students and their problems. One particularly was worrying us. He was a third-year student from the Oicha pre-rebellion school, clever and capable. IIe worked hard and was obviously determined to do well. There were periodic 'troubles' in school, as there will be in any large group of senior teenagers – student pranks that go too far; minor disobediences that nearly end in disaster; strikes over the time-tables, or the food, or some such current problem – but Hezekiah kept apart from each episode, determined not to be involved in any insurrection. We were conscious, however, that he was not really pulling with us. I almost felt he despised me, for working with the students on the buildings, for talking colloquial Swahili more fluently than the official French, and for being a foreigner and a woman at that!

About eight miles out from Nyankunde we drew to a stop at the roadside, under a large mango tree. Two students scrambled down, clutching Bibles and hymnbooks, and a pile of tracts and Gospels. The rest of us moved on towards Irumu, as the two pushed their way up the narrow track leading through the waiving maize to a hidden group of round huts, to gather children and adults together for a service. Just before Irumu two more students got off, at a long lane of thatched houses winding down into the valley, full of laughing children, goats and chickens, and various wary adult spectators. On again to the Irumu prison, with its twenty or thirty inmates. They were mostly ex-Simbas, largely in their late teens or early twenties, all bored and disillusioned, and glad of the interruption to prison routine, even at the price of singing a few hymns.

Two more students stopped at the hospital: two at the further outskirts of Irumu, near the army camp. We continued into the country, over the river, up a steep, winding hill, to a group of houses in a wide plateau of maize fields. Here we called a halt at what we came to know as 'our village'.

Honking the horn as we approached, we watched the children come running from all sides. A youth started to beat an old iron wheel-hub suspended from the beams of the palaver hut. The village elder came smilingly across from his home carrying two dilapidated chairs (the very best he had) for his 'honoured guests'. Handshakes and greetings all round, chatter and laughter, as slowly some sixty, or even eighty, folk gathered, it would seem miraculously, from nowhere. All were largely naked or clothed in torn tatters: they sat on branches or on the dusty ground: and they listened intently.

Hezekiah led the worship and he was excellent. He seemed to enter right into the lives and thoughts of the people, and talked as one of them. Jill gave her testimony that first week, in Swahili, and I remember how thrilled we were that we had gone. We went regularly after that first Sunday, and began to get to know the villagers.

Twin boys came regularly, sometimes in shining white T-shirts and little red pants, sometimes just tied around with a scruffy piece of cloth. An intelligent little eight-year-old girl always sat on the front row, with her small sister, and drank in all that went on – the hymns, the reading, the message and prayer. In two weeks she was singing the hymns by heart, her whole face lit up by an inner happiness.

One week, as the assistant student was preaching, her little sister, uncomfortable on her bit of the tree trunk, punched the little girl next to her, pushed her off and took her place. The second little mite, dirty as they come, with a filthy cloth round her, lifted up her head and howled dismally. Hezekiah quietly slipped across, picked her up in his arms, slipped back to his seat and sat and soothed her. She sat through the rest of the service in his arms, her head nestling against his chest trustfully and silently. That little act of loving sympathy, where another would have slapped the child, or told her firmly to be quiet or to get out, spoke more to the congregation of the reality of the gospel of love that we preached, than even the words we used. We thanked Hezekiah on the way home, and found that we *were* pulling together, after all!

Then there was our first Christmas. We had only two months to prepare an 'item' for college participation in the festival services. By then we had fifty young men but only three girls in the student body. What could we sing, and whom could we inveigle into helping us as sopranos? We wanted something definite, to mark the first Christmas of our Training College, to involve us all and to glorify God. It should be sufficiently difficult to demand hard work and some sacrifice regarding time, if it was to be of any value as part of the curriculum, yet simple enough to be well executed, if it was to be truly part of the worship of the congregation. We chose the Hallelujah Chorus of Handel's *Messiah*.

We had sung this before, at Nebobongo, at Christmas in 1961, and I still had our tonic solfa rendering and Swahili version. Practices began in November. Qualified and pupil midwives agreed to join us, as did also three of the European nurses. A time had to be chosen to suit both groups from the college and from the maternity unit, and these had to be during daylight hours, as the church lighting system had not been restored since the Rebellion. So we fixed rehearsals each Wednesday afternoon at 1.30 p.m. The first week I turned up, armed with tuning-fork and blackboard already covered with solfa-hieroglyphics for the first page. I waited. By 1.45 p.m. a few had wandered in. By two o'clock there were about fifteen, and my patience was wearing thin. At last we started, and did fairly well for an introduction.

Next week, despite all our urging, the start was equally delayed. They appeared to remember very little of what we had previously studied, until I realized that they had all swapped places, basses deciding to sing alto, and tenors preferring bass. We started all over again, dividing them into four voices and taking their names to prevent too much changing in future. While I was teaching a section to the sopranos, the altos and tenors started chattering. Silencing them, we started again, and then several late-comers arrived and had to be sorted out into their places. I asked the altos to sing their part alone and a somewhat unmusical 'cat's chorus' resulted: the sopranos all roared with laughter. The male students were deeply offended and almost refused to try again. The basses, bored by the proceedings, were doing homework, and failed to respond at all when their turn came.

The practice finished in grim silence, and I left in glum frustration. During the following week I painstakingly typed out stencils and duplicated one hundred copies of the Chorus with the tonic solfa. Next week, most arrived on time, waited in uneasy silence, sang as demanded – and it needed half an hour to win their co-operation again and persuade them to *enjoy* the exercise instead of only suffering the agony. Slowly it took shape. I pressed for more practices – after evening studies; after lunch; each voice separately; in various groups. Time was running out. We were far from perfect. Could we really do it? Was it just a publicity stunt on my part?

Christmas Day dawned bright and clear. The students marched across to the church in their well-pressed Sunday uniforms, singing hymns, to the accompaniment of trumpets and drums. Slowly the church filled with a capacity crowd of 1,500, and many more outside the doors and windows. There was community carol singing, special items from different groups of primary schoolchildren, two good messages on the wonder of the coming of the Christ to redeem us from our sins, and then, as a glorious finale, the college was invited to sing the Chorus. It was beautiful and very moving, especially knowing all that had gone before in the preparation. A great hush of wonder settled over the whole congregation, who had never heard such music before, and one sensed that all hearts were lifted and filled with praise to God. As they finished, there was a long, silent pause that eased into a shuddering sigh of satisfaction. For us, it had made our Christmas complete and memorable.

At the end of that first term, in mid-January 1967, Jill and I filled the ten-day school holiday with a rapid and exciting trip back to my old hospital at Nebobongo. The seventeen hours' driving to cover the 350 miles, mostly in sunshine, were accomplished with practically no difficulty. At one road-barrier, where a soldier was checking my driving licence and stamping all our road-passes, a discontented chicken started loudly protesting. The soldier then demanded road-passes for all our livestock. We just managed to suppress our laughter, and assured him that we had only one chicken which was to be tomorrow's dinner. Eventually we persuaded him to accept our plausible explanation.

Florence Stebbing, my colleague through the eleven years' work at Nebobongo, had arrived back that same week, on her return after the Rebellion, and she had hardly had time to settle in before we turned up. Daisy Kingdon, one of our veteran missionaries, was staying with Florence, as it was considered unwise for any foreigner, especially a woman, to be on her own at that time. Colin and Ina Buckley, missionaries from Isiro, were also there, with two tons of supplies to help the hundreds of destitute refugees still pouring out of hiding in the forest to the south.

When Jill and I drove in, unexpected despite letters and

telegrams (which eventually arrived after our departure), at 9.30 p.m. in the dark, the house which had previously been my home for many years seemed almost uncomfortably full. Camp-beds were everywhere, and bales of blankets, cartons of drugs and sacks of foodstuffs were stacked along all the walls. If our quarters were cramped, however, our welcome certainly was not! The unbounded joy of our Nebobongo team that I was back among them, even if only for a week, was very moving.

The week sped by. A visit to Ibambi to deliver stores that we had brought from Bunia turned into a busman's holiday, with a crowd of a hundred really ill patients to be seen. Then we went to see their new maternity-unit. Senior midwife Martha Anakesi had been responsible for its construction by the husbands and friends of her clientele. It was spotless in its fresh whitewash, and filled to capacity with contented mothers and babies. This visit was one of the highlights of our week. It was a great encouragement to me to see something of what the African staff could achieve on their own, and to know that we had had the privilege of some little part in their training.

Two days were given up to journeys to Isiro, the local township 40 miles north, to do essential shopping for food and stores; and to Egbita, another church centre some 40 miles north-east, to do a clinic for the sick and to examine eyes for reading glasses.

Our two Sundays were filled with 'missionary activity', preaching to a packed church, Bible study with the nurses, fellowship meetings with the church elders. As always, the abandoned happiness of the singing of the Christian family caught at my heart, and I realized afresh how much I was part of them.

Then five packed days of doctoring. Everything had to be included. One day included four hours in the leprosy-care centre examining fifty-two new patients and checking over one hundred others, writing up their report cards, checking on drugs and dosage schedules, and generally encouraging them. Another day we arranged a clinic for the eighty primary schoolchildren, checking teeth, eyes, skin, blood and stools, looking for anaemias, due to intestinal worms or chronic malaria, leprosy or tuberculosis. Yet another day we spent many hours in the pharmacy, cleaning, re-arranging, listing, making up quantities of stock drug mixtures and injection solutions, and a list of urgently required replacements.

When we had arrived, everywhere had seemed a little dilapidated and rather dirty. Thieves had broken in the previous week and taken all the operating-room linen, quantities of penicillin and vitally needed drugs, syringes and instruments, and the African staff were somewhat discouraged and depressed. The stores and enthusiasm that we brought with us did much to restore courage and replenish shelves. Everyone set to, with scrubbing-brushes and disinfectant, sewing-machine and rolls of cloth, firewood and sterilizers, and the operating-theatre was soon transformed into its usual dignity. Seven drums were packed with new cloths, gowns and gloves; three small autoclaves were all hard at work; floor, tables and trolleys were spotless; rows of instruments, trays and catgut had all been sorted into four general sets; and we were ready to start!

We managed five major surgical cases each morning, mostly hernias and fibromes, with a couple of emergency Caesarian sections. Afternoons were given to clinics – tuberculosis cases, leprosy patients, schoolchildren, eye diseases and those needing glasses, as well as regular outpatients' clinics with chronic malaria, undernourishment, intestinal worms, all complicated with severe anaemia. Each evening, a ward-round to see some fifty very sick patients. Only the most seriously ill came to hospital, as their abject poverty made even our heavily-subsidized fees seem exorbitant. How we longed to do more for them, but how? and with what?

An incident occurred during our visit to Isiro, which somehow illustrates the problems of black/white relationships of that period. I had ordered a 40-gallon drum of petrol, and entered the shop to pay for it. While I was there Jill hurried in to tell me that the drum had fallen on to the toe of one of the helpers and that 'the toe is half severed off!'.

I'm afraid Jill was surprised that I did not go at once to see the man, but instincts, developed during eleven years in

Congo, restrained me. I turned to the shopkeeper and reported the matter to him in Swahili. He at once went to see, and I delayed a little longer in the shop. Then we went out and saw the shopkeeper standing on the kerb, arms crossed behind his back, four assistants working hard in sweating silence to load the drum on the trailer, and then to fill the four jerrycans and tank. Glancing round I saw the 'bystander' two or three yards away, squatting, holding on to his bleeding toe, and scowling at the shopkeeper. Jill urged me (fortunately in English) to go and see him. I gently pushed her away towards the van. Gathering our shopping-lists and handbags, and locking the van doors, I guided her away from the scene to do our other errands.

'Why?' she asked. 'Aren't you a doctor? How could you possibly leave him? And he was actually *helping* you when it happened!'

I tried to explain what might occur if we became involved, thus revealing that we felt responsible, which would be interpreted as guilty – a court case, two or three days' delay, insurance claims, lots of unpleasantness. I assured her that I was willing to give the man all he needed to be taken to the local hospital, but that I was not responsible: and that in 'these days' it would be very unwise for a white person to be involved in an accident in which an African was injured. Jill remained sceptical and was not too pleased with me, and I wasn't too sure in my own heart just how plausible it all sounded.

Ten minutes later I went back to the van with a load of groceries, to be met by two policemen with open notebooks, and we were quickly surrounded by an interested crowd. Fortunately I remained outwardly calm, though the fear, born in the Rebellion, was nearly stifling me. Asked for an explanation of the 'broken toe case', I said the least possible, stressing the financial element in the knowledge that in African law this would absolve me from direct responsibility.

'I had *bought* this drum of petrol, which was being loaded on to my van by the shopkeeper's workmen, when this bystander apparently came too near and was hurt. Actually, I wasn't present at the moment of the accident as I was in the shop *paying* for the petrol and labour.'

Fortunately the police (and crowd!) were satisfied, and turned to the shopkeeper.

'I'll willingly examine the man's toe, if you wish it,' I offered to the policemen, 'and drive him to the hospital should this be necessary.'

They assured me that this was not necessary; that they would see to it directly themselves – and they thanked me for my 'generous offer and obvious concern'. We left, and I couldn't blame Jill for the look of scorn that I had so easily accepted such undeserved praise; yet we were deeply relieved that what might have led to considerable unpleasantness had ended so peacefully.

Jill and I wanted our home at Nyankunde to be African in style, a home where Africans could always feel at home. We wanted it to be like our school buildings, so that there would be as little difference as possible between us. We wanted it to be made almost entirely of local material, by village workmen, so that Africans might be encouraged to build equally good homes in their own villages. It had to be within our income, and yet pass the fairly strict standards set by our local building committee.

The European family had asked Jill and me to consider building a duplex (two-in-one semi-detached bungalow), and by January 1967 the housing situation was sufficiently urgent to ensure that when we presented our plans to the building committee, they were passed with very little opposition. We were delighted!

We tramped over the hills to the south of the hospital and college, to choose our site. Higher up the views were glorious, but the land very exposed to the strong easterly gales: lower down, it would be much easier to reach the site with building materials, much closer to the college for supervision, but we would sacrifice some of the views. We timed ourselves clambering up and down from college to various sites: we cleared small patches, spent an afternoon at each, studying and reading, and eventually we picked a site to the west of the main valley, 'half-way up', really 'neither up nor down'!

Once again, in mid-January, when we presented our plans

in greater detail, including the site and direction and drainage, we were thrilled that they were passed at once. On Monday 6 February four workmen started clearing the site; eight went to local afforestation areas to cut poles; others went farther afield for grass for thatching before the annual burning of the fields in early March. Yet another group went daily to dig out sand and gravel from various pits in the vicinity; and we began to watch the materials arriving.

Every day we would go up to the site to see how things were progressing, but it seemed such slow work. The ground was rock hard, and digging out a site from the mountainside really demanded great effort, especially with our very primitive tools.

At last the site was levelled to take our 40-ft by 26-ft bungalow. Then to drive 2-ft-deep holes in the rock surface to take the poles, four main supports of 1-ft diameter, sixteen other supports of 10-in. diameter, and then almost 300 for all the framework poles of 8 in. diameter – what a task! Hands were blistered, one crowbar was broken, several pickaxes made useless before the job was completed.

Meanwhile others had cut poles to the right length, prepared the top end in a forked notch to carry the ridge-poles, cleaned and prepared ridge-poles for the five main support-lines.

The first week in April was a school holiday for Easter, and so, early on Tuesday morning at 6.30 a.m., Jill and I joined the work force, and watched as the wall frames suddenly went up. Then the sixteen subsidiary supports; then the four main central supports – eucalyptus trees, straight and strong, almost 24 ft high – hoisting them slowly upwards, slipping their bases into the prepared pits, fixing them upright with forest-twine pulleys on all four sides. Quickly the workmen roped scaffolding branches 2 yds high to hold the whole framework in position: standing on these, another circle of scaffolding $3\frac{1}{2}$ yds high completed the preparation.

On Wednesday we hoisted the ridge-poles. The outside wall ridges first; then scaffolding across the house at ceiling level; then the formation of a 'human scaffold', five workmen to each side of each of the four main support-poles, each standing on another's shoulders. It was an amazing and somewhat frightening sight to watch as we hoisted the main central ridge, a 40-ft-long eucalyptus trunk, up the human chain of scaffolding, from ground to outstretched hand, up to shoulder level, up again with outstretched arm to the down-reaching hand of the man above. Students stood around and a great silence fell as the huge pole slowly rose, and rose, and rose into the blue sky. All necks stretched back, eyes glued to the pole. The slightest slip by any man would have been disastrous. The final pushing upwards by the fifth team of eight men; the straining of every muscle . . .

'It's up!' – a cheer went up, as bated breath was released.

The roofing timbers went up quickly in the following week. Then the whole roof was closely covered with line upon line of strong stalks of elephant-grass, bound on with forest vines.

Others were preparing grass. Twenty-four tons had been carried in. It all had to be cleaned from bracken and foliage: gathered in lengths, tied in 2-yd-long bundles 6 ins. thick, and then cut in half. Bundles were neatly stacked all round the house. Coiled lengths of split vines were soaking in water-butts.

Amazingly, the dry season held. Rains were two weeks over-due. Each morning the sky was filled with dark, lowering clouds, but they blew away by midday and the building pro-gressed.

The slope of the roof, at almost 45°, scared the local work-men. Basuana, from the northern forest region, was accustomed to it, but they were unwilling to believe him that it was really safe. So I took a day off school, and scrambled up and sat astride the top ridge to encourage them when they started the thatching! This seemed to go very slowly: methodically set-ting the first line along the lowest edge, with the cut end to-wards the ground and the long, loose leaves up to heaven, and binding each bundle to the framework; then line after line, binding on to alternate rows of elephant-stalks, patiently, accurately, knotting the soaking vine; twisting and knotting, twisting and knotting, slowly moving around the house, line upon line. At last it was complete, except for the final ridge.

Then bundles of longer, uncut grass were thrown like jave-lins from ground to ridge, and bound on strongly astride the ridge. The next night it poured with rain for five long hours!

This firmly beat the thatch into place. After three such storms another row of grass bundles was attached astride the ridge. After yet further storms a final third row was fixed into position and the roof was secure. Probably 18 tons of grass were up there, held by a few forest trees, tied down with thin twists of split vines. It seemed incredible that this could hold up against the fantastic tropical storms, gale-force winds and thundering rains. The thatch was 15 ins. thick when completed, and planned to last a probable ten to twelve years, before needing replacement.

Sheltered from the rains now, as the seasons changed, and working under the roof, a framework of thin branches or bamboo stems was attached horizontally outside and inside the pole structure, to all the outside and inside walls. We were into May when 'mudding' started and the wall-framework was stuffed with mud, smeared with mud, plastered with mud. Then it was left for two weeks to dry out before a final plastering inside and out with mud mixed with cow-dung, which set hard like cement.

Window-frames and door-frames, prepared by a local carpenter, were set in. Water was brought to the home by pipes from the hospital water-supply system, and Richard Dix, a missionary construction engineer in charge of the over-all building programme at Nyankunde, gave us bathroom and kitchen taps and toilet. Cement floors were laid, doors were hung, walls were whitewashed, windows were put in. The outside was swept and cleared, and flowers planted – and by 30 June, Independence Day 1967, we moved in!

It really was exciting to be in our own little home. A local carpenter had made us some lovely bedroom, dining-room and office furniture, all in grained red-wood. Curtains had been measured, cushions prepared, rush mats for the sitting-room acquired – and we were in, five months from starting to clear the ground. True, another month was needed to complete the small garage and cookhouse behind the bungalow, levelling the drive, clearing up the garden, but the job was completed in and around all the regular duties of lecturing and administration and hospital practice.

As our first school year drew to a close and Jill and I had a moment to assess the situation, various pointers prompted us to make a trip to East Africa. First, we urgently needed equipment for the new college laboratory, both for the first-year orientation classes in elementary physics and chemistry, and also for the third- and fourth-year students in medical procedures, requiring microscopes and chemicals. Secondly, my father was planning to visit us for a week and hoped we could meet him in Kampala and drive him back to Nyankunde. Thirdly, there was growing unrest amongst the troops in the National Army, with disturbing rumours of the possibility of an attempted coup to restore Moise Tshombe to power.

We packed up a minimum of supplies for the journey and set off early one morning, at the start of the long summer holidays. We travelled in the Land Rover with trailer, and took with us two Africans who had not previously travelled outside their own province, Basuana Bernard and Gandisi Benjamin. As we crossed over the great central mountain range at 8,000 ft, from Zaire to Uganda, and dropped down the escarpment to the east to the source of the Nile, our two African colleagues were tremendously thrilled. The motor-driven ferry across the Nile; the hundreds of enormous elephants calmly munching at the water's edge, eyeing us disinterestedly like ruminating cows at home; the thundering water at the Karima bridge near the Murchison Falls, with spray thrown up to form a fantastic rainbow arched across the valley; these impressive sights drew exclamations of wonder.

Walking up the streets of Kampala, a pleasant tropical town to us Europeans but an overwhelming city to our African colleagues, completed their amazement. The shops, the traffic, houses of several storeys, Indian temples, the lights at night, the airport and the arrival and departure of great planes with over a hundred passengers each ... the days were not long enough to satiate their curiosity.

We acquired the laboratory and other school and household equipment we had come for, and packed the van and trailer to capacity. We met my father and started the long journey back to Nyankunde, going through the National Park to see the Murchison Falls in all their glory.

Then followed a lovely week, in our new home which had been finished only two weeks before, but all the time we were nervously listening to radio broadcasts indicating the worsening situation and danger in our area. I must confess that I was glad when the week was up, and we set off for the border again before trouble broke. Once out of the country, into East Africa, I could relax and enjoy the long trip to Nairobi from where my father flew on to Malawi.

Jill and I spent a week camping near Nairobi before going to the Kenya Keswick Convention, where I had been invited to speak about our experiences in the Simba uprising.

Then the long trek back to Kampala, as the first lap of the journey back to Zaire, only to be checked by a request to visit the British High Commissioner. He asked us not to proceed to Zaire at that time, as the situation was so uncertain and they feared a fresh outbreak of hostilities.

Frankly, I was pleased to be stopped by Authority. I feared to go back in. I had had enough in 1964, but I didn't want the responsibility of making the decision. Jill was champing at the bit to get back to the job at Nyankunde, and must have found my easy acquiescence most irritating, especially as I was the driver and she was entirely dependent on me for transport.

We were not the only ones 'shut out' at that time, and we soon met other missionaries. Some had just got out with great difficulty from farther south, due to the mutiny of the mercenary troops serving under General Mobutu. Others were on their way to Zaire for the first time and were understandably hesitant. We all waited for a green light from the British High Commissioner.

Meanwhile, to fill in time profitably and to try to prepare for the new school year ahead of us, we visited the University library for several days. We then travelled to the eastern border of Uganda to Mbali to visit the medical auxiliary training school there, to study their programme and course material. After a week there as welcome guests with the headmistress of the local girls' school, we journeyed back to Kenya and spent a wonderful month on a farm of friends of my father, whom we had visited a few weeks earlier. The holiday was a real refreshment, with plenty of time for reading, writing and preparation for the new school year.

At last, impatient of receiving no news, no letters, no word from the Embassy, we set out on the journey home and made an uneventful entry! There were no difficulties at the border, no customs duties to pay on our few purchases, no accident to the van, in fact nothing worthy of report at all. We drove into Nyankunde late on Saturday evening, hoping to start school on the Monday, and what a welcome awaited us! One would have thought we had been gone a year, instead of a month or so. Apparently that Sunday had been pin-pointed as D-day. If we were not back, all senior students were to be sent home, as the remaining staff felt they simply could not cope with all three classes, as well as all their own hospital and dispensary responsibilities.

Students poured out of the village and we were mobbed. Laughter and singing, crying and clapping. Missionaries seemed to arrive from every direction, and our hands felt limp from shaking, before we eventually reached home and settled back into routine for a new school year.

Chapter 8   1968-1970
Seeking recognition

After my visit to Kinshasa in May 1966, it was obvious that one of the very basic requirements, if we were to gain Government recognition for our college, was that we should have permanent buildings to 'specified standards'. It was almost impossible to discover what these standards were: some said one thing, some another. I gathered that a certain cubic metrage of air per student per class-room was demanded, which was an interesting requirement in the wide-open spaces of our mountain site! Internal flush-toilets had to be included, even though the students would have to be trained in their use, never having met such things in their village life. Obviously the building would have to be constructed in permanent materials, and this posed plenty of problems, compared to the simplicity of putting up our own small home.

We decided to tackle first a class-room block with auditorium, laboratory, library and administrative offices; and later, to construct a separate dining-hall with kitchens and food-stores. Many and varied plans were prepared and studied and turned down for one reason or another. Eventually a very simple plan of a 130-ft-long building, 40 ft wide, with a long central corridor and rooms along both sides, was found to be the most economical as well as the most useful plan. The completed building would be four times as large as our home and would probably cost eight times as much. Richard Dix, the builder attached to the hospital, was basically in charge, but he had an enormous building programme in hand for the hospital and staff homes. So he agreed to allow Basuana and myself to tackle the job of school construction under his supervision. Eventually the necessary permission was granted by the local building committee and we started to prepare the site in June 1968.

Fifty thousand bricks were available, from a newly-built kiln that Richard had completed. Six tons of cement and 500 sheets of corrugated asbestos roofing were purchased. Louvre window-frames and glass were ordered.

Twenty-four workmen were employed in four groups of six, each group with a semi-qualified mason in charge, assisted by a villager who showed enough intelligence and initiative to be trained as a mason, and four locals for digging trenches, carrying bricks, making mud, and generally helping to complete each team. Basuana had the immediate oversight and direction.

The land was cleared and levelled; then Richard came, complete with instruments, to lay out the foundations. Basuana was fascinated! He and I had always squared our corners with the old three-four-five measurements and pegs, checking with equal diagonals, and making sure that all was level with a spirit-level laid on our strings. *This* was quite different, efficient and accurate, and Basuana drank in every detail.

Then the digging of trenches, while others quarried huge stones from the mountainside near the local river. The trenches were filled with stones, carefully laid and levelled in concrete. Then the four groups separated to the four corners, and the walls started to creep up. Between classes I used to rush over the half mile from our temporary school quarters to the new building, to check on corners and levels, bonding and mudding. Students used to rush over in break, and stand around in the dinner-hour, to watch. Everyone became excited as the gaps for windows began to appear. Then window-frames and door-frames were bolted in. Then reinforcing irons and concrete slabs were laid all round the structure, and a further five lines of bricks brought the huge building to ceiling height.

Students would wander round inside in the evenings, trying to decide which room would be what, and getting a real thrill as they were allowed to help on Saturdays to speed the work along.

The dry season came and we were ready to put the roof on.

But here we paused. Basuana and I had never tackled so large a building before, and we felt that we just could not manage a roof of such dimensions. Richard's workmen, under his supervision, had prepared the triangle trusses for us, and all was ready; but Richard had several other urgent tasks on hand and simply could not spare the time to put the roof on yet. So we started praying that the Lord would send us a 'roof-er'.

Meanwhile we did every conceivable other job that we could find. Richard sent a plumber over to help us prepare for putting in the water-system. The masons got ahead with pointing the whole building. The carpenter hung doors and fixed window-frames. The workmen carried gravel for preparing the floors for cement. Still no 'roof-er'.

We squared the corners of the roofing; we stacked the triangle trusses in place around the building; we carried sand for plastering the inside walls; we prepared timbers for surrounds under the eaves. We even cleared away all debris, smoothed the paths, planted grass and flowers, and cut a giant eucalyptus for flagpole. Still no 'roof-er'.

One Thursday evening in January 1969 Basuana came to me.

'Shall I dismiss the workmen and tell them not to come tomorrow? There just isn't another job to be done, and there's no point paying them for doing nothing.'

We eyed each other. We had worked together for fifteen years and just about knew the thoughts going through each other's mind.

'No,' I said, grinning suddenly. 'No. Let's trust for the roof tomorrow.'

'O.K. by me,' and we let the matter rest.

That night I was woken by a car coming up the hill, and peeped through the curtains to see if I was needed. No; the car drew up next door, at Dr Ruth Dix's house. Lights went on and I could hear voices. Shortly I saw Ruth leave and drive down the hill to the hospital. I prayed for her that all would be well, rolled over and went back to sleep.

Next morning, going down the hill at 6.20 a.m. to prayers with our workmen, before starting school, I passed a young American going up the hill. I greeted him and he nodded, but looked too weary to bother to speak. Suddenly Basuana came running up towards me.

'Do you know who that is, that you passed on the hill?' he panted excitedly. I didn't.

'He's a roof-er!' – and as I realized the import of these words, the two of us turned and hurried back up the hill.

'Sir,' I called out breathlessly.

He turned politely, if with a puzzled look.

'Please do excuse me, I don't even know your name, but is it true that you're a roof-er?'

'I beg your pardon?' he said in a confused way. 'I'm Ruscoe Lee, but I don't quite understand what you asked me.'

Hardly surprising! We explained our situation, and he explained his. He had driven in during the night to be with his wife Rachel, who had been flown to Nyankunde the previous day for urgent hospital care under Dr Ruth Dix's supervision. And he was a roof-er! During Rachel's two weeks of care and convalescence, Ruscoe worked hard with the African team and achieved our goal – the roof on!

There still seemed so much to do, though. Ceilings, electrical wiring, plumbing, flooring, plastering, painting – the jobs seemed endless. Then furniture began to arrive: forty desks and forms, fifteen tables, 180 chairs, cupboards and shelves. All had to be sandpapered and varnished. Blackboards had to be plugged to the walls. Laboratory equipment, pharmaceutical scales and drugs, nursing arts' teaching models, charts and library books: all had to be listed and put in place.

Then in May 1969, at the annual meeting of the Board of Directors, we had the college officially opened, singing the National Anthem, raising the flag, cutting the red tape, and we were truly launched. The service, the speeches, the choir, the thanksgiving feast all soon became items of college history, but the sheer joy of teaching in good and adequate premises is a permanent present-tense reality.

Before the college building was finished, the Inspectors had arrived! Since classes had started in 1966 we had kept Kinshasa in touch with us. We regularly sent them progress reports of every part of the Nyankunde programme. We continually put together what we considered necessary for a 'dossier', despite great ignorance as to what was really needed. Local educational authorities were loath to help us, as we were under the direction of the Ministry of Health rather than of Education. Now and again I'd catch a hint of a better way of presenting our material and at once we would re-compile the whole dossier, typing out several copies and sending them off to all the authorities which we felt might be even remotely interested in us.

For over a year we heard nothing from Kinshasa. Then someone passed us a verbal message that applications for recognition must go first through regional channels, then provincial, before approaching central. With unflagging willingness we started all over again, and actually achieved regional 'consent', for what it was worth. I rushed off to Kisangani, the provincial centre, clutching the regional letter of recommendation and all the carefully-prepared copies of our dossier.

A week of dogged perseverance followed. I went back to the same office twice a day, till eventually the provincial medical director was persuaded to give me an audience. Most graciously he added his signature to that of the regional authorities, and suggested that I go next to the Governor of the Province (as he was then styled).

Another week of equally dogged perseverance, only at the last to be told that I had broken etiquette by going to the medical director before the Governor

'The Governor will not look at a document already signed by a subordinate. His signature authorizes medical and educational authorities to continue with their investigations into the suitability of the application.'

Back to square one. Another set of documents was rapidly prepared and taken to the Governor, who graciously signed them. Back to the medical director, only to find that he had just left on a six-weeks' tour of the interior. Over to the director of education, and roughly the same procedure through another week till I found him in, and willing to listen; but it took several more visits to persuade him to take action. Even then, he would not sign our documents till he had had time to send an inspector up to see our standards.

I flew back east to Nyankunde and got back into school routine, teaching some twenty-four periods a week with all the preparations involved, as well as office administrative procedures. Everything was made ready for the promised inspector; no-one came.

At the start of a new school year, in September 1967, we actually received a specimen document from Kinshasa as to how to apply for recognition. We speedily re-prepared our ever-fattening dossier according to this newest formula, and sent off three copies to the address specified.

We waited in vain for an acknowledgment from Kinshasa.

We waited in vain for an inspector from Kisangani.

We sent letters of request to both. Eventually Kinshasa replied that they had never received our dossier. We did it again and sent it off by registered mail. Two months later, it was returned to us with a cryptic message that we deciphered to mean that we must submit our papers through the right channel.

What was the right channel? We sent to the local regional authority, to be told that their jurisdiction did not extend to para-medical schools. We went to provincial authority, to be told that they could do nothing till our previous papers of application were duly completed and signed. We reminded them that we were waiting for an inspector, only to be sharply told that this was now quite unnecessary. I promptly produced my earlier forms, carrying the Governor's signature, photostat copies of the medical director's signature, and the space waiting for the educational authority's signature.

He actually signed – and I sent them all off the same day by registered mail to Kinshasa, accompanied by our precious dossier.

Three months passed by.

In May 1968 the papers all came back, without the dossier, saying these forms were now obsolete, and would I please procure and fill in the new forms for requesting school recognition?

Where did one procure such forms?

Teaching and preparation continued.

In September, we received a new application form. Somewhat automatically we filled it all in, re-did the dossier, affixed

130

all the end-of-the-last-year reports, and all the beginning-of-the-new-year reports, and sent everything off.

Teaching and preparation continued, in our cramped temporary buildings, while every effort was being made to speed the construction of the new permanent building.

Rumour reached us that inspectors were on their way. We tried to school ourselves to ignore such rumours: they only built up to frustration and disappointment. Yet one day they would prove true, so we did all we could to prepare. All student dossiers were checked and brought up-to-date. All didactic material was listed and catalogued. Our Swiss staff put in overtime to check and correct the French of our course material.

The inspectors arrived! In November 1968, one Tuesday afternoon, the Government doctor from our neighbouring town of Bunia drove out to us, with two European ladies (a Yugoslav and a Britisher) accompanying a Zairian from the Ministry of Health at Kisangani. This was it!

That first afternoon, in a continual drizzle, pushing our way through mud and rubble, we set off to inspect the new school building, then up to ceiling height (and awaiting its roof!). It was the biggest building I had ever been involved in and I sometimes felt guilty at its size, in those days of economic uncertainty. Would we be able to complete it, and would we really have enough students to fill it?

The national inspector asked endless questions about the size of each room, the lighting, ventilation, electricity and water supplies and sanitation arrangements.

'My one criticism is that it is all too small. The minimum size of a class-room of a secondary school has been set up by my Government as 48 square yards, or at least 5 cubic yards per student.'

I did some rapid calculations, quickly making a mental note of each room and its proposed usage. I then led him down the central corridor to the first- and second-year class-rooms, where only the foundation was in for the dividing-wall.

'Will not this satisfy the requirements?' I queried, motioning to the one large, undivided room, 11 yards long by 5 yards wide. He paced it out, and no more was said. We never built the dividing-wall. Honour was satisfied on both sides, with no loss of face.

Up to our temporary mud-and-thatch village, through the two dormitories, the dining-room and cookhouse, the home of a married student with his cookhouse and toilet facilities. The students hadn't been warned: would they rise to the occasion? And anyway, could anyone really think our village satisfactory? Even in my own heart, proud though I was of the students for having achieved this village and being willing to wait for better accommodation, I knew that this was little better than the proverbial 'shanty town'.

'I think this is wonderful,' one inspector commented. 'All local materials to meet local needs, within the local economy. Very commendable!'

Was I really hearing aright?

'And the rooms are so clean and tidy: a real credit to the college.'

Boys, thank you!

We moved away, through the hospital compound towards our temporary school buildings. By now darkness had descended, and the students were in the class-rooms studying. We went first to our tiny office, where I tried to interest the inspectors in the filing system and the students' private dossiers, but they were obviously tired and not interested.

Next door, the five senior students were studying. All of these had been in our Nebobongo school before the Rebellion. They were older men, most of them married, and some with very rudimentary French. Before the Rebellion much of their teaching had been in Swahili, and I had not worried overmuch about this aspect when they came to complete their schooling at Nyankunde. The two ladies were watching them and making towards them. I tried to edge them away and into the large first-year class-room, where we had a crowd of keen teenagers with good French and an ability to express themselves. Un-successfully!

Moving into the fourth-year class-room, the inspectors started to ask the students questions about public health, the care of the tuberculosis patient according to the latest proposals of the World Health Organization, and I licked my lips in apprehension. Joel looked across at me, in hopeless bewilderment; Lawi was turning the pages of a book, at least knowing where to find the answers; when suddenly Gaston saved the situation, sailing into an excellent extempore dissertation on the care of the tuberculosis patient. There may have been some wild guesses; there was certainly some very original thinking; grammatical howlers filled every phrase; but sheer enthusiasm for the subject of preventive medicine could not have been more abundantly portrayed if they had been schooled to it.

We did eventually enter the first-year class-room, where students were painstakingly copying down a very elaborate diagram of the interaction of hormones in the control of the health of the body. Their notebooks were beautiful. The blackboard diagram was the pride of my heart.

'This is absurd – quite outside the scope of the curriculum and of no possible real value to the work they are going to do.'

I felt like a deflated balloon. The national inspector had to leave us to return to Kisangani, and I was left to the mercy of those two highly-qualified, high-powered, W.H.O. lady inspectors.

The next two days were agony. They grilled me. Nothing seemed to please them. Mostly we sat in our sitting-room going through course materials and programmes, while other staff kept the school time-table going as best they could. The subjects that the inspectors were keen on were those that I knew practically nothing about, such as the growing importance attached to the teaching of preventive medicine and public health. The subjects I knew best, and loved teaching, and had spent patient years developing, were to them of minimal importance, such as basic anatomy and physiology, the science of diagnostic medicine, the principles behind the surgical procedures we employed. We just didn't seem to have any common ground. The more they talked and reasoned and explained and instructed, the more I felt that I was on a different wavelength, and had been altogether wrong in my whole approach to the establishment of the college and its standards.

Was the whole college, as I had envisaged it, only an outworking of *my* vision and individuality? Had I really felt I knew just how it should be done and, if they would let me, I'd prove to the Government that I was right, until they would actually turn and thank me, even would eventually adopt my plan and method? Had I allowed some basic inborn feeling of white superiority to drive me along, irrespective of what the local Government was demanding? Was I really training a new generation to be discontented and maladjusted, because their courses would not fit them to take their place in their developing country? Would they really feel underpaid according to Government salary structure, because I had taught them too much for a junior diploma?

Could I really be all that these inspectors implied?

It certainly was a terrible blow to my pride. I simply couldn't face the enormity of the consequence of these allegations: all I could do was to pack and go home. What a fool I'd been, what a proud, stubborn fool – and I really had dreamt I'd be thanked for all my effort, or, at least, I'd be satisfied by the worthwhileness of all that was to have been achieved.

By Friday midday I could take no more. I broke down and cried, and asked them please to stop. 'Better you talk to the other staff. They'll be more able to adapt. I've just made a mess, a proud stupid mess. I'll leave. The others will know how to benefit from all you're saying.'

My house-help, Benjamin, unable to understand as we talked English, and hardly better able to understand when we used French, could easily understand atmosphere and now tears. He was furious that these two strangers had so upset 'his' doctor, and tore off down the hill to the school to collect Jill and Liliane.

Meanwhile the two inspectors were equally horrified. Whatever had they said to upset me? 'But of course, the college is *wonderful*. It is one of the very best that we have seen in the country so far.'

But why on earth hadn't they said so before?

'But our job is to show you the one or two areas where it could be improved.' Liliane and Jill arrived at this point, followed by an almost savage-looking Benjamin, who was quickly dispatched to prepare coffee and biscuits all round. And we started again.

By that evening, the two inspectors had had a meeting with

the students to encourage them, and to promise them that everything possible was being done to acquire the coveted recognition, and that, meanwhile, they had a college to be proud of. They had also a meeting with all the staff together, to present their final findings and to promise us that they would recommend us for immediate recognition and, following that, for upgrading to the status of a senior technical college. Furthermore they had a meeting with all the missionary personnel of the Medical Centre, and explained again the great importance of close co-operation between hospital and college, the need to increase our bed capacity to 250 as soon as possible, and our qualified nursing personnel to a minimum of one to every fourteen beds, more than double what we had at that time.

On Saturday, Jill and I went out with the two ladies for a picnic, to the escarpment overlooking Lake Albert. It was a lovely, still, hazy day, and we enjoyed chatting about one thing and another, nothing to do with the college, until it was time to take them to catch their plane back to Kinshasa.

Arrived back at the college, we were immediately surrounded by students.

'Did it succeed?'

Did what succeed? We looked puzzled. Everyone talked at once. At last we made out that the student body presumed our 'outing' for the day was in order to bribe the ladies to give us what we so dearly longed for. We were tempted to roar with laughter – the whole concept was so completely foreign to our very English way of doing things – till we realized how utterly serious they were. This is what we should have done, as our students saw it; and if we failed to become recognized now, it was indeed our own direct, wilful fault.

And it was to be two and half years before we heard any more. That 'fault' was going to cost us dearly.

The first real indication of growing irritation among the students came during the final week of the 1969–70 school year, eighteen months after that inspection. Nothing had apparently come of it, and so, in frustration, the students staged a revolt against the staff: minor, perhaps, but no less traumatic.

They were impatient with their Government for not providing legal diplomas. These had been virtually promised for June 1970 or so I had said. They hadn't materialized. Had their Government failed them, or was it possible that I, school director but foreigner, had lied? Had there perhaps never been an agreement, and was it all my bluff, to – to what? To satisfy my 'neo-colonialist' instincts to make them do what I wanted? Or to satisfy my 'imperialist west' plan to achieve cheap labour for the hospital that we foreigners were running? Such were the thoughts fed to the students daily over eastern radio broadcasts. Perhaps they were true after all?

Anyway, it was easier to strike out against local known leadership than the far-distant unknown Government, so we had to take the brunt of their frustrated dissatisfaction.

We were within a week of the final oral examinations. Petty irritations began to occur in all classes. Students came in late with no apology; others deliberately sat when answering questions, where the custom was to stand. Some refused to make any attempt to take part in discussion groups; all of them seemed suspicious and sullen. We had a meeting in the assembly-hall to try to heal the breach before the fuse blew, but we got no co-operation. Eventually one asked to see the diplomas that they were going to receive at the end of term, and with an almost audible sigh of relief we felt that we had discovered the root of the trouble.

Knowing that they would be disappointed that the official documents still had not come (weren't we all?), we had had new diplomas printed locally. They were as near to the coveted Government ones as we dared to approach, using the same format, but keeping our college name and crest in evidence, and our motto clearly printed at the base: 'The Son of man came not to be served but to serve, and to give his life a ransom for many.'

I went along to the office and collected one of each of our college documents – diploma, certificate, report card, annual bulletin, as well as road-passes and student passes for reduced rates on public transport. Back in the hall, staff and students awaited my return in strained silence. I showed each document in turn, beginning from the last, and briefly explained both its value and also its format. When I held up the diploma I was booed. Everyone started talking at once, and in the general hubbub I caught phrases:

'Why on earth is there a Scripture verse on a diploma?'

'What value has that piece of paper, with no Government signature?'

'Who's going to sign it, anyway?'

'How dare you imitate a Government document?'

'Who do you think you are, anyway?'

At last the noise exhausted itself, and I briefly answered some of the criticisms I had managed to distinguish from the torrent of angry comment.

'We have written permission from the Government to produce our own diplomas again this year . . .' angry booing interrupting me as I spoke; '. . . so long as we show clearly that it is not in fact legal,' and the angry shouts drowned anything else I could say.

'Listen, fellows, give it a chance. The exams are on Tuesday. If the examiner comes as promised, if the exams are fair and you pass, if he stamps these diplomas with a Government-recognized seal and duly signs them as the Government-appointed official, won't that content you?'

Obviously not, as the torrent of noise increased again and ugly looks were being exchanged.

'I promise you that I have done all that I can to get the official documents here, and I won't cease to go on badgering the Government till they come' – but my words were silenced in mocking jeers of 'wretched impostor', 'imperialist white' and 'it's all been a hoax'.

On Saturday morning I received an anonymous, badly-written, poorly-worded, scruffy letter on a sheet torn from an exercise book. We called their bluff and sent it back for signature. Triumphantly they returned it with all but four of the senior students' signatures.

On Sunday I carefully answered the letter, point by point, in polite, accurate French on college notepaper, explaining again all they already knew.

On Monday both sides watched each other warily, and no-one moved.

Tuesday was our big day. Staff had worked hard all Monday to prepare the library for the visiting examiner, to prepare the questions for the oral examinations, to prepare diplomas and certificates to be duly filled in as each student completed his quarter-of-an-hour oral, so that all would be ready for signature and stamping at the end of the four-hour session. On Tuesday morning fresh flowers were placed on the table, trays for mid-morning coffee prepared, students alerted as to their order and practical details for the smooth running of the day: and we waited.

Promptly at 8.0 a.m. the Belgian doctor from Bunia drove in, alone. We had expected a Zairian doctor too, but we accepted the change philosophically. He worked hard and efficiently. The exams were quick and fair. Every student of second- and third-year classes successfully passed the required 60% mark. Diplomas and certificates were filled in, checked, signed and stamped according to recognized international custom. And the doctor left us shortly after midday.

Normally all the students would have been in the assembly-hall to greet the examining doctor and hear the results. Then speeches would be made by both sides, and considerable freedom of expression allowed to let off steam. That day the hall was empty, no-one came to hear the results, no-one thanked anyone. With some embarrassment the staff saw Dr Marchand off and sincerely thanked him for his services and time.

Turning back into the shool, we sensed the gathering storm but met no-one. We cleared up and went home for lunch.

Then they came, a fairly small group at first, climbing the hill in silence. A last, fleeting hope that they might be coming to thank us for their schooling was quickly squashed as they lined up outside our small verandah and angrily shouted abuse at me. Two held batons menacingly. All looked hard and disagreeable. It was inconceivable that these were our own students, our friends, for whom we had cared, whom we had clothed and taught for the past four years. Their threats were sinister, using gestures and vocabulary learnt from the Simba rebels, and therefore even more frightening to my ears.

Through various stages, up and down the hill, they besieged our little home for the next twelve hours, and we were, quite

138

honestly, scared. They sang lewd songs, they threatened us and shouted abuse at us, they threw stones at the doors and windows . . . but that was all.

Next morning, no students reported to the hospital for work. There should have been twenty-six of them, in the six wards, outpatients' department, laboratory and operating theatre. There were none. Graduate staff, foreign and national, worked round the clock and saw that the patients did not suffer. Letters went to and fro; conciliatory offers were made; veiled threats were returned. Eventually at 4.0 p.m. they agreed to meet with Dr Becker as arbitrator, on condition that he went alone. Normally one would never question 'going alone', but even the tone of voice in which they demanded this was calculated to strike fear in my heart.

Then it all fizzled out. By the end of the week all the ringleaders of each class had left for summer vacations. Those who were prepared to sign a statement of compromise stayed on to work in the hospital. Diploma day and festivities were all cancelled, but not before the staff and the four senior students who had refused to sign the original protest had all had their fill of insults and threats. The students suffered worst: their property was seized and fouled, buckets of water poured over their beds, everything they owned rendered useless.

It was perhaps only a petty show of frustration, as some tried to persuade me, but it left a dark stain in my heart. When I drove the first group to Bunia to put them on public transport for their various destinations, all at our expense, they had spat at me – and that burnt deep. Oh, granted that they were only students, and did not really represent the general feelings of the population; nevertheless they were *our* students and it mattered to me tremendously what our relationship was going to be in the future.

The very next week, at the end of the first half of our projected eight-year programme, I left for England for a quick three-month holiday. I needed a breathing-space to look at things from a distance so as to assess the real situation. Also I wanted a short time with my mother, who had been ill during the previous two years. She had spent many months in hospital, having operations on both her knees, and was then limited to two crutches and a wheel-chair. While on holiday with her in Cornwall I weighed up carefully whether I honestly wanted to face the students again.

What was being achieved? Were our results worth the price that was being paid? As I looked back over the twelve years of my medical career at Nebobongo, where I had been a full-time doctor – surgeon, physician, obstetrician and pediatrician all rolled into one – I asked myself again: 'Is it worth giving up all *that* for *this*?' That is: giving up being in charge of a medical service for the problems of running a training college to staff such a service.

Many of my close friends were quite sure it was not worth such a price. Yet I remembered times at Nebobongo, too, when I had seriously questioned if being in charge of a medical service was worth while. At first, when I found myself so involved in building, and buying food stores in the market, and caring for orphan children, and developing the student nurses' school, that there was no time for being a doctor, I had grumbled.

Eventually I had been persuaded to see that all these activities had brought me nearer the people. When my hands were raw with throwing newly-burnt bricks down from a kiln, the workmen understood and accepted me as one of themselves; whereas when I was drawing on sterile surgical gloves to operate on a seriously ill child, I was a thousand miles away from them, on a pedestal of respect and awe. When I fumbled around in the Kibudu language down at the markets, the village-folk roared with laughter and loved me; whereas when I was teaching in school in French, even the students held me apart as an object of discipline.

Later on, when I found myself so overwhelmed with medical responsibilities, endless surgical emergencies day and night, hours needed in the pharmacy for making up accurate solutions of drugs, time spent in the laboratory coping with tests and analyses beyond the ability of our students, so that there was no time for being a missionary, I had grumbled. Eventually our evangelist Agoya had persuaded me to look at things differently.

'Listen, there are 300 people coming to our hospital daily. Why are they there?'

I wasn't going to be drawn.

'Because *you* are here! If you, the doctor, weren't here, they wouldn't come. And what do you think *we* are doing?' Agoya and his wife Taadi were both Bible School trained evangelists, and Basuana and his wife Andugui were catechists, appointed by the church to full-time ministry in the hospital.

'All day and every day the four of us are fully occupied talking to patients in the clinics, the wards, the health centres. Do you realize that five, ten, sometimes twenty people are finding Christ as their Saviour every week through this ministry?' He paused, and then added quietly: 'You know, Doctor, we can't all be the last link in the chain!'

My thoughts moved on to the recent four years at Nyankunde. I never did surgery now; I hardly ever entered the wards and only rarely helped in outpatients. The students did not respect me as a doctor, but merely tolerated me as a teacher. Even my teaching ability was now in question and was to become more and more so in the three years ahead. I was becoming an office-boy rather than a teacher, let alone a doctor. Was this reasonable or worth while? Did this really make sense under the title of a 'medical missionary'?

Someone else was to take over first-year teaching, including anatomy and physiology; another the youth club and sports activities; another had been nominated to represent the school on the executive medical committee of the Centre which handled school disciplinary problems. More and more, I was to sit and type out seemingly hundreds of Government forms, adding up seemingly endless columns of figures and statistics, filling in seemingly useless reports and documents.

Why? Was something really wrong? Had I made a mistake, and somewhere got out of the line of the Lord's will? Basuana, on our school committee, had tried to talk sense back into me during the previous year.

'Listen, Doctor; think for a moment of Cornelius, and Isaac, and Bernard, and Mordecai; cast your mind to Poko, Aba, Nala, Oicha, ...' and he named a whole list of college graduates, and the places where they were then working.

'How many graduates from our college are now in full-time church employment, do you think? And how many patients are they reaching daily, not only with medicines and also with the gospel?'

I knew what he was heading towards without doing the calculation; however, he wanted an answer.

'Well, I suppose some forty graduates so far, and they're working in twenty-two of our hospitals and dispensaries, and so I suppose they are seeing at least 3,000 patients daily, and might be even more – and that is not counting the thousand patients daily here at Nyankunde.'

'O.K., and how do we come to have these graduates?'

I thought back quickly over all the trials and tribulations of those first four years at Nyankunde, all the staff and workers involved, all the preparations, teaching, demonstrations, as well as office work that had achieved even our present position.

'You know, Doctor, the Government demands a doctor's signature on all the forms and letters to authorize the very existence of this college. And really ...' and he used the same Swahili idiom as I had heard years before at Nebobongo from Agoya: 'we can't all be the last link in the chain.'

As I remembered all this and reviewed things from the perspective of the cliffs of Cornwall, in the quiet peace of a summer day, I let the impatience in my heart simmer down, and I made arrangements to go back to Zaire at the end of the month and to carry on.

Chapter 9   1971-1973
Recognition at last!

Without doubt, the Government was grateful for all the funds channelled into its medical services from overseas by private agencies, including the enormous contribution made by the missionary societies, but they could hardly be expected to take this into account when planning a new national health service. We also had to realize that a country's self-respect cannot accept endless voluntary contributions, especially if these are in danger of dictating policy by their very largeness in comparison to the national effort.

So we were not altogether surprised when a move was made to change the pattern. Almost out of the blue we heard that our application for Government recognition of our college had apparently been (or was about to be) granted, and so the country's treasury had been authorized to pay a subsidy towards the salaries of the four registered, qualified teaching staff. With this short notification came four pay-sheets, and the assurance that the money mentioned could be withdrawn immediately from the local bank.

Rather exciting, even if the cheques were small compared to homeland equivalents: about £60 a month for our nurses, £80 for the sister-tutor, and just over £100 for myself as medical director. I wrote at once to all those who by their sacrificial giving had kept our college going during the five years since the Rebellion, to let them know that the Government intended to carry one-third of the responsibility in future. This would be increased by increments until they could economically afford to accept the whole budget on the national grid.

Accordingly a certain degree of overseas support ceased. Simultaneously the Government-promised aid failed to materialize. Hadn't God known the latter when He agreed to the former? There were a few 'light' months with hardly enough to pay the workmen. Then came the long summer vacation, when college feeding-bills and running costs reached their annual minimum and we maintained par. However, these same months usually included stocking for the coming school year. Tons of rice, beans, groundnuts, dried fish, flour, sugar and palm oil: thirty local-made beds with mattress covers and blankets for the new first-year students: uniforms, stationery and class-room supplies all needed replenishing.

I had been ill in February of that year with a mild attack of tick-borne typhus fever, and the rather severe depression that followed this made it advisable that I should go home to England for two months to regain strength. At home, on holiday, I made out lists of all our college needs; I prepared lectures and time-tables; and I tried to rest and relax, rather than chewing my nails over the enormous, unresolved problem of turning my paperwork into practical realities.

I arrived back at Nyankunde on the first day of September with four days before the college was due to re-open. On my desk, amid a mountain of mail, was a statement from our regional educational authorities of a gift of almost £1,500! – unsolicited, entirely unexpected, and probably unprecedented. Doubtless God had already arranged this provision when He allowed other sources to dry up temporarily. Even after twenty years of experiencing His unfailing faithfulness in such matters, and His amazing accuracy in timing, I still had not managed to accept the period of uncertainty with equanimity.

Now, with this generous gift in hand, we went the next day to Bunia and turned all the prepared lists into acquired realities, and then found we still had sufficient funds in hand for the first quarter of the new year.

Despite repeated efforts to correct our Government pay-sheets, my own remained obstinately at just over £20 a month for several months, and then stopped altogether. The following April I, along with others, attended a teach-in at the regional educational offices in Kisangani, some 400 miles to the west.

It proved to be an excellent and valuable, if intensive, three days, dealing mainly with various financial aspects of our service. This included how to fill in forms to apply for subsidies for salaries, equipment and didactic material, and then how to fill in more forms when the response to the first set was not satisfactory.

During one session, the national lecturer told us of the dubious excitement being enjoyed at that moment due to the installation of a vast new computer to handle all national grid salaries for the armed forces and police, the telecommunication service personnel, educational, medical and general transport personnel. He explained a little of the vast programming involved for each service, to include basics, educational bonuses, family allowances, transport and lodging expenses, all deductions for pensions, national tax, health services and others. He explained how the punch cards were prepared from statistics provided, and the checking system employed before the final feed-in ticker-tape was actually ready. With all this, he indicated some of the thousands of possible hold-ups or pitfalls. Finally, various listings would reach regional, and then sectional, sorting offices, post offices and banks, for distributing to groups of services, through to area representatives, and so ultimately to the individual.

Pinpointing some of the hazards of the system, and how easily mistakes could get in but how hardly they could then be got out, he told us a story.

'We have a medical doctor as a director of one of our secondary school extension programmes, training medical auxiliaries. The punchcard code is DD, but when the computer met this for the first time, it queried it as a mistake, and so substituted D6. When this came through, the computer realized the error, as D6 would mean a secondary school director with only six years of secondary school education, an impossibility in our revised educational system. So the code was duly changed to d6, temporary director with six years of post-primary education: and the salary came through at about £20 a month. After a few months the computer caught up with its error, that a qualified medical doctor was earning only £20 a month, so it cancelled the pay-sheet and fed it back into the machine for correction, including back-pay. By now this totalled over £600. The computer had been taught that any monthly pay sheet over £500 must be an error, so again the result was cancelled and fed back in.'

Amid growing amusement as the story unfolded, the lecturer further explained that this school director had thus received nothing at all for several months. He looked across at me then and grinned, concluding: 'I confess I'm glad she's white, or she would doubtless have been on strike these months, living on my office doorstep, till we could sort out the computer!'

The school year 1971–72 went remarkably smoothly until the last month. As usual, an application had been made to the central Government in February for a Jury to be formed in June for our finalist students. Hearing nothing, we wrote again in April. As there was still no acknowledgment or response, we telegraphed Kinshasa in May. In the first week of June we received a telegram asking if we wanted a Jury that year or no, and if so, when. Frantically we sent an answering telegram, and also an unofficial verbal message by radio. The examinations were due Tuesday, 12 June. We had one week left for arrangements.

We had a radio message on Thursday, 7 June that the central Government had authorized the regional authorities to make all necessary arrangements, and they were glad to delegate their authority to sectional level. Would I therefore contact Dr Biki, the national Goverment doctor at our local hospital in Bunia, and also the inspector of secondary schools at the local offices of the Ministry of Education, to arrange details?

We set off, on what proved to be a long trail. Dr Biki was not in. The Educational Office said that it would agree to whatever Dr Biki suggested for Tuesday the 12th. Dr Biki was not found in at all on Thursday the 7th nor on Friday the 8th. On Saturday, I managed to waylay him as he left his home in the early morning.

'No,' he said emphatically. 'I certainly cannot accept delegated authority by word of mouth. There must be written confirmation.'

Back to the post office to send a telegram to Kisangani, and to sit there four hours waiting for a reply. They were about to close at midday and I was growing frantic. Eventually our local post office relented and allowed me to use their radio-telegram line myself, and I contacted the head postmaster at Kisangani. Understanding the urgency of the situation, he agreed to send a runner round to the Ministry of Education and to radio me back in half an hour.

I sat on by myself in a now-closed post office, not even sure if I knew how to let myself out, let alone how to handle the radio, telegram and telex machinery.

Two hours ticked relentlessly by, and I felt it was a wasted job. I might as well give in, and return on Monday morning. I put my things together, turned off the machines, went to turn off the lights – when a sudden hunch made me try once again. Switching on the machine, I called in Kisangani post office, and they replied!

'We're doing all we can for you. A telex has been sent to Kinshasa, as the Provincial Medical Director who nominated Dr Biki as his delegate is away, giving examinations at Isiro, and we cannot contact him. We may hear by 5.0 p.m. and we'll radio you.'

I had to be content. I went back to tell Dr Biki this news, and he nonchalantly started talking about the examinations. Had we set the questions yet? Yes? Good, he'd like to see a set. Oh, you've got them with you? Excellent. Thank you very much.

He started flicking through the patiently prepared lists of thirty questions in each of twelve subjects.

'Have the students seen these?'

'Of course not,' I exclaimed.

'Why not? You must show them to the students at once. That is only fair.' You couldn't win with this man.

I went back to the post office and waited till six o'clock and tried unsuccessfully to call Kisangani several times. At last I gave up and went home. Monday found me back at the post office as soon as it opened. There was no telex, nor telegram, nor letter. Nothing. Eventually we established radio contact with Kisangani.

'We're doing all we can. We have no contact today with

Kinshasa. We have sent copies of all telex of the weekend down on this morning's plane. We'll radio you as soon as we hear anything.'

Time was running out. The date set for the examinations was tomorrow. I managed to contact the missionaries in Kisangani by radio and asked them to get anyone possible from either the Ministry of Education or the Ministry of Health to their radio by 11.30 a.m. to rendezvous Dr Biki, and so give him the needed authority to act. I rushed off to persuade Dr Biki to come to the radio; but he refused. Back by myself, I spoke with the Kisangani authority and explained my difficulty to them.

'But we *have* sent Dr Biki a telegram nominating him for tomorrow's Jury.'

'Please, can you send another, *now*, and I'll stand by for its delivery and take it out to him.'

'Certainly.'

I stood by till the office closed at 4.30 p.m. No telegram. What could I do next? I went back to the Ministry of Education. The inspector was ready for the following morning and obviously irritated by the unnecessary fuss. I retired. Eventually I decided to spend the night in Bunia. Early Tuesday morning, I contacted Dr Biki at his home.

No, he had heard nothing.

No, he was not willing to act without proper authority.

I went back to the Ministry of Education, where the inspector shrugged his shoulders.

All day, I hovered from one to the other. Eventually at 4.30 p.m. there was a telegram for Dr Biki. No, the post office would not give it to me to deliver. No, they had no runner available to take it: it must wait till tomorrow. No, it would be no use my going for Dr Biki, as they were closing.

I felt frantic, when suddenly Dr Biki himself appeared! He took the telegram, read it, and brusquely said: 'All right, we'll have the examinations on Thursday, 8.0 a.m. Be ready!' and swinging round, he left. I rushed off to the Ministry of Education, but everywhere was closed: all the personnel had left for home. I'd no idea where they lived.

Once more I drove home and told everyone the news. On

Wednesday I drove again to Bunia to be sure the Inspector of Education would be available for 8.0 a.m. Thursday, and to arrange for his transport.

'I'm sorry, Miss. The inspector leaves today on the plane. He has other examinations booked elsewhere tomorrow. No, he hasn't left any instructions. No, nor has he left his rubber stamp.'

How could this happen? I stopped short as I realized that I was running round in ever-narrowing circles. I took a grip on myself and had a short time of quiet prayer.

Then I set out again. By lunch-time I had persuaded the Ministry of Education to send a primary school inspector to us. They had discovered the needed rubber stamp, and contacted their senior authority for permission to use it. I had the address of the junior inspector and knew where to find his home.

After lunch I went back to Dr Biki to ask if his chauffeur could go to pick up the inspector at 7.0 a.m. and bring them both to Nyankunde by 8.0 a.m. for the Jury. I gave the address, and started on the explanation as to how to find the place.

'Over in the suburbs? Good gracious, no! My chauffeur is not going over there. Why hasn't he got a car of his own? If he must come with me, he can walk into the city.'

I was furious. The sheer snobbery, that 'we of the city' were a superior class to 'them of the suburbs', left me dazed. I knew this sort of thing back home among Europeans but I'd never met it among Africans.

'Please don't worry. I'll come in for him myself tomorrow morning.'

I turned to leave, when Dr Biki called me back. Picking up the copies of the examination questions lying beside him, he leisurely tore them across and delicately dropped them into his waste-paper-basket.

'Those are useless. No good at all. We need clear, simple questions on each subject, such as . . .' and for ten minutes he rattled off suggestions. I grabbed a pencil, dipped into the waste-paper-basket for a torn remnant, and scribbled as fast as I could.

'Oh, and my chauffeur will collect your inspector tomorrow,' he threw at me as he finished.

I left him, seething inwardly at my own impotence. I was sure this had just been an idle show of power to put me in my place, but it all seemed so unjust, so unnecessary. I raced the thirty miles home, tore round to collect all the staff up to my home and explained the situation to them. Then we all worked half the night preparing new questions, typing sheets and re-arranging things to fit in with the last-minute suggestions that Dr Biki had given.

At 8.30 a.m. they arrived and a grim day started. Nothing pleased him, nothing was right. Why ever didn't I know how to organize things better? At Kimpese they had done it this way – or that way – but never my way! Contrary to custom, he asked questions in the main, instead of the staff, and many students could not even follow his rapid French. They were all so nervous. Many questions were far too hard and simply not geared to our syllabus. He argued with the staff over almost every answer given. We felt the day would never end; yet as each student stumbled out of the room in a daze, Dr Biki wrote down a mark on his report card, invariably higher than any member of staff would have given. No student failed.

At last it was over. All certificates and diplomas were filled in. Augusta Johannessen, an elderly Norwegian lady who had been living with me all the year and tirelessly serving the school as our secretary, had everything ready for Dr Biki to sign within a few minutes of the last student leaving the library. Then the next row started.

He certainly wasn't going to sign anything. He had only been asked to witness the examinations. If Education wanted to sign, that was fine by him. No, he was adamant: he would make his report to his superiors, as to just how unsuitable the examinations had been, how poorly organized, how 'altogether-wrong'. He then strode into the hall to face the rows of dazed students, waiting in bewildered silence, to hear the end of the strange day. He faced them all belligerently, and swung round to me.

'Where's the list?'

All was ready, Sir. Here at once, Sir.

And he read out, to the dumb-founded college, the amazing list of 100% unqualified success. After an unbelieving pause, the whole student body burst into cheers. The senior student made a good quick speech of thanks, to which Dr Biki replied with extraordinary graciousness.

The following school year, 1972–73, started off quite normally. The previous year had been a good one. Mordecai Kasereka had been an excellent head student and diploma day had been a happy occasion for us all.

There was a large new first-year intake, including six girls. We were under pressure on all sides to take girls, to give them two years' general nursing training, and then a third year concentrating on midwifery. The whole north-eastern region, with a population of some five million, was urgently needing qualified midwives, women who could not only undertake responsibility in rural maternities for the care of normal deliveries, but also the care of complicated cases. Since the Rebellion it had been hard to recruit girls: there were not many in our secondary schools, and all who reached a sufficient level in general education seemed to want to go on to university, to prove their equality with the boys.

For the first time we had four girls who had finished the two years' general nursing training and were admitted to the third year to train as midwives. The staff spent considerable time and care planning their course and time-table, to make it not only efficient and practical, but also attractive. There were not really enough of us on the teaching staff to carry a four-year programme, and so considerable doubling of classes had to be manoeuvred. Third-year women midwives and third-year male medical assistants could follow almost half their programmes together with very little difficulty, and each would benefit from the extra material given to the other.

We had four weeks' preliminary training school with the new first-year students, while second- and third-year students had their annual vacation, and during this period the main preparation was done for the school year for all four classes.

In October we started full classes, with all third-year students, men and women, in class, and second-year students working on the wards. We were excited and expected a good year, with enthusiasm for the new courses. Application had been duly made to the Government to recognize our midwifery section, as our nursing and medical auxiliary sections were already accredited.

From the start we found it heavy going, to say the least of it. By the end of four weeks, all the staff were tired of encouraging, persuading, cajoling the third year to work and study and co-operate. They simply wouldn't. A sort of don't-care attitude pervaded their class-room. Slowly it became clear that the girls were the ringleaders. We invited them home to coffee and cakes, to share with them more informally our hopes for the success of the year's programme, and their prospects as the first qualified midwives under the new Government plans. But no response. No enthusiasm.

Another staff member invited them out. Every effort was made to 'get through' to them, and eventually someone tipped us the clue we needed. I sent for them again.

'Someone tells me that there is an absurd rumour going round that you will not get diplomas of equivalent value to the men's.'

Silence.

'You know of course that this is rubbish. They are identical in value.'

Silence.

'Are you worried about the salary-scale at the end of your training?'

No answer.

I produced copies of both finalist diplomas for third-year studies. I produced the Government wage-scale for para-medical workers, male and female. I produced the law-book, controlling para-medical training colleges, course materials and programmes.

No response.

I nearly lost patience, and told them to stop wasting their time and mine, to start working and putting their backs into their studies, to pull with the rest of the class, and to help us all to make it a good year.

They left, unimpressed – and school continued under strain.

Another hint reached us, so we tried again. All the staff got together and invited Dr Ruth Dix, the obstetrician in charge of the maternity unit, to join us. We discussed together, prayed together, and then invited the four girls to join us for coffee and cakes, in a relaxed atmosphere.

'Have you any questions you'd like to ask me, about the syllabus this year, or the opportunities for service next year?' Ruth asked them.

Vague indifference; monosyllabic answers.

'You know how much we are looking forward to having qualified help in our maternity units. I'm prepared to do all I can to help you to get all the skill and knowledge possible, to rise to the top of your profession.'

Polite agreement; nothing more.

Studies dragged on interminably, with none of the usual joy and fun. Quite honestly, we all became a bit bored with the effort of winning their confidence or trying to help them. Petty disobediences, frequent late arrivals, unwillingness to do any public service such as cleaning the school and grounds on Saturday mornings, refusal to attend church or weekly fellowship meetings, uncooperativeness at choir practice: all this harassed and aggravated us.

Then, during the ten-day Christmas vacation, the storm began to burst. A letter was written to Dr Becker demanding student representation at executive level. A meeting was called, and the students produced a list of some twenty demands, mostly involving pay for practical service in hospital during their training, redistribution of hours of service giving more to theory and less to practical, the right to know what staff did with their Government salaries and a continuing angry demand to know why we were not yet a legally-recognized college with Government diplomas.

Each demand was answered as reasonably as possible. All the staff managed to remain calm and polite, even in the face of outrageous demands touching their own salaries. Students were allowed to examine the books, to see the Government pay-roll and the Government schedule of distribution of hours for theoretical and practical teaching – all of which they had seen before; but every effort was made to satisfy them.

They tried to threaten that they would not work in hospital unless they were paid. The whole executive committee balked at this. Every student was being heavily subsidized already for schooling, housing and clothing. Their practical work was part of their training. We all gave our hours voluntarily to teach and train them. Anyway, there simply was no money available to pay them.

'O.K. then, we won't work,' was the student ultimatum.

'O.K. then, we don't teach,' was the staff rejoinder.

Stalemate. I left the room. Why continue? We, the staff, did not need them, the students. We owed them nothing, but were willing to give them everything, as I saw it. Until qualified, they did need us, however unpalatable the truth might be. I was almost tired of serving them as a slave, with just no response at all on their side.

The students went back to work.

The staff returned to teach.

But the tensions in the class-room increased rather than eased.

Classes were to divide after Christmas, girls having their own programme, practical and theoretical, until Easter, and the men theirs. That was when we finally found the underlying cause of friction. No girls turned up to their practicals; they all came to the boys' instead, and they came in a militantly aggressive way as Mrs Pankhurst of the English suffragettes might have done!

'We will *not* be treated as inferior to the fellows. We are equal. Give us our rights. We intend taking the same courses, the same exams, the same diplomas. We are equal.'

To suggest that to attend their own courses showed their superiority, as the men were not invited to be midwives, was to court disaster. The four militant female students were in no mood for reasoning. They had made up their minds – or rather, their minds had been subtly made up for them – that the only way to show their equality with the male students was to force this particular issue. We soon discovered that they had been systematically brainwashed during the first three months of the school year, over the radio. Broadcasts in French from Kinshasa, broadcasts in Swahili from farther east, had been repeating day after day that the women of Zaire must insist on their rights, demand absolute equality, refuse to be made out less than their male counterparts.

At Christmas, the final thrust had been made over the Voice of Zaire radio network.

'Girls in Medical Auxiliary Training Schools! Don't let your staff tell you that you can only be midwives! Don't listen to their specious reasoning why it is better for you to be a midwife than a health officer! Demand your rights! Fight for equality!'

And our four were going to fight!

We didn't give in easily. As we assured them, it was for their own good that we did all we could to persuade them to do midwifery. They were needed as midwives by the population.

'Isn't the first object of our political leaders that we should serve the people?'

As midwives, they would have jobs assured, but no-one would employ them as health officers, as we couldn't send a woman to a rural village on her own.

'Are you threatening us? We'll report you to the Party!'

And they meant it. And we didn't like it – and they knew it!

So they joined the men's classes. We closed the midwives' class for the year. We sent a report to the local Government doctor and the educational authorities. The year crept on much as it had started, with a veiled campaign of passive resistance, no co-operation and less-veiled glances of contemptuous superiority.

However, the truth remained that we urgently needed qualified midwives, and that African culture made it strongly preferable for our girl students to train as midwives rather than as health officers. Ultimately we, the staff, felt sure that these same girls would regret the action they had taken. So we made plans to ensure that this would not occur again. At the end of term, when reports were to be given out, each second-year student was asked to sign a request form to be admitted to third-year studies subject to their exam results; and the men's form, all made out in the masculine, requested entrance to 'the health officers' course of studies', while the girls' form, written with feminine concords, requested entrance to 'the midwives' course of studies'.

We sent for the six second-year girl students, explained the whole situation to them again, and gave them their request forms to sign. Forms were in duplicate, so that they could send a copy to their parents or to their local Party member, should they so wish. No pressure was put on them. They could sign and do midwifery, or not sign and go home. As simple as that. There was no option open to the girls to sign for the health officers' course. We merely stated that the latter course was already full with sixteen male students.

We waited. One girl went home without signing, to 'discuss it with my father'. Three girls came up to see us to 'talk it over more fully'. Staff were nervous: students were edgy. The local Government doctor, who had initially backed us and given us his authority to take this course of action, withdrew his support, and warned us that we might be heading for trouble with the Party.

At four o'clock one Tuesday afternoon there was a knock at my front door.

'Good afternoon, Doctor. This is my father and brother,' spoke a second-year girl student, indicating the two visitors she had brought up the hill.

'Good afternoon,' I responded, and we all shook hands.

I suggested to the girl student that she go back to the girls' quarters, while I talked to her parent. I turned to go in and make them tea.

'No,' the father snapped. 'She stays.'

I paused, took a deep breath and turned to face them. The very air felt menacing. Then a mud-slinging contest started, voices were raised, tempers became heated and I knew fear. I had no witness, no-one to quote me accurately, no-one to defend me against the outlandish accusations that this man was making against me. I knew fear of direct physical violence, that he would strike me, and I knew I dared not defend myself. I knew fear for the college, that, after all we had done to establish it, one foul slander from this man could lose us our Government recognition. It was all so weird, so unreasonable. It was useless to reason with him: he had already decided on his course of action before ever he approached me. He was almost demented, beside himself with rage.

At last, others came and took him away, talked with him and appeared to reach a conclusion. They went, and I breathed a little more easily.

Two days later a letter came, a copy of a letter of bitter accusation that this man had sent to the judiciary powers in Bunia, to the special powers that controlled the movements of foreigners and held our dossiers, to the Party and to the National Army. He claimed that, as a foreigner, I was acting for a foreign power, against the best interests of Zaire, that I had ridiculed the Party and the Flag, and that I had stood in the way of his daughter receiving the best possible education provided by the Government, showing sex discrimination and anti-Party colonialism.

The case dragged on for nearly three months. Several times I had to appear in court in Bunia, costing not only £5 each trip, but also several hours of precious time. Reports were written and submitted, explanations were prepared and given, advice and consultation on all levels was sought and received. Lumbabo Eugène of our educational office was a tower of strength. He knew the right people to give us the legal help we needed, particularly with regard to court-room custom and language. He gave me his friendship and time without measure. He represented me several times, when he felt that an African could cope better than a foreigner. His report to the court officer on my reputation and relationship with local Africans was generous to an extreme.

Eventually the affair 'blew over', or was allowed to settle. I was acquitted, I presume, although no-one quite said so. Some-one would have lost face had that been done. Those three months of court appearances and uncertainties were almost like the proverbial straw that breaks the camel's back. Not one word of appreciation from this parent for all we had taught his daughter; not one word of apology for his cruel lies and absurd accusations; not one word about reimbursement for all that the court case had cost me. No, but next term he was to come to Dr Becker and ask the medical staff of the Centre to employ his daughter in the hospital, as though nothing had ever occurred!

Despite Government salaries for the staff and a Government doctor for our final examinations, we still had no paper to say we were truly recognized and accredited as a Government college. We needed a legal identity number to put on all our Government communications. We needed a formal statement with a clear signature to say that the Government had agreed to our request for recognition. We still had not received any Government diplomas for our graduating students with which they could obtain official posts with recognized salaries in the Government health service. All we had was the salary for four foreign teachers. In the eyes of the Government this was our personal money and we were not expected to account for its use, only to sign for its reception. If in fact we each ploughed it all back into the running expenses of the college, this was our own private affair and of no account to the Government, however grateful they might be for what, to them, must be obvious generosity.

The students heard that we had received Government subsidies, and so they concluded that the college was recognized. This should have meant that the college was also receiving direct subsidy money for the use of the students, but this was not yet so. The facts were explained to the students, but they chose not to believe us. The only alternative was therefore to believe that we were lying, hiding from them the truth, presumably (in the thinking of the students) because we were stealing the college subsidy for our own private use. They were shown the books and the Government-salary pay-sheets. Members of the district educational office explained the situation to them patiently and in considerable detail. Still they could not, or would not, believe what we said: and a growing spirit of criticism and suspicion crept in between staff and students.

We applied repeatedly to the Government to have some Africans on our pay-roll. True, we had no national with full teaching qualification available for our school staff, but we had some fine young men, graduates of our college, who stayed on at the Centre to help train first-year students. Their main responsibilities were in the realm of the art of nursing (bed care and ward routine) and to control discipline in class-rooms and dormitories. We felt that, if even one of them were on the pay-roll, students would be more likely to believe them than at present they were to believe us, when only foreigners were paid.

In October 1972, to our delight, three Africans were added to the pay-roll. All seven of us, black and white, went each month to the local educational offices to receive our 'salaries' and sign for them. Everything was open; each one could see what the other received; and we hopefully expected the underground mutterings and discontent and suspicion to subside.

What a vain hope! By Christmas, while women students fought for their rights, men students clamoured for cash. Their conviction appeared to be that the Government money we were accepting as our salaries was meant to be their pocket-money! At their request (as I have mentioned) I showed them my monthly pay-slip, totalling about 32 Zaires (£30), on official computer form. They were dumbfounded, and yet still not convinced. True, they did not know that my salary-subsidy was so low due to a mistake in the computerization, but even they must have sensed something a little bizarre, when a qualified doctor with over twenty years' experience, director of a training college, was receiving the same as one of the college graduates with only two years' experience.

For six months the undercurrent of grumbles and suspicions rumbled on, periodically flashing into the open. I was ill for five weeks during February and March, and to make up to the students for all the lectures they had missed in that period, we offered to rearrange their time-tables. It would mean very heavy hours for the staff, perhaps especially for myself, but very little ultimate change for the students. However, the third year representative student came to see me to refuse categorically all the changes we had suggested, unless we paid them 'for the inconvenience'.

It was almost incomprehensible to us as a staff. Our African colleagues tried in vain to reason with the students, to show them that only they would be the losers: the staff were not sitting their final exams! To the students, apparently, it was equally incomprehensible that we were willing to put ourselves out for them with no ulterior motive. They refused to believe it possible, convinced that we were putting something over on them. They sent us their suggestions for the final three months of the school year, with an apparent ultimatum stating what they were willing to do if we did not pay them for their services.

We accepted their suggestions, just as they stood. It meant far fewer teaching hours for us. We determined among ourselves to carry the extra hours of practical service in the hospital, rather than make any further appeal to the students.

Then suddenly we heard that the scholarship grants were on their way!

We heard a vague, unofficial report that these grants were to be paid to individual students, and not to the college as previously indicated. Then we heard from a school in Kinshasa similar to our own, that they had received their grants. The next week we heard that violent trouble had broken out in that school due to a misunderstanding of the use intended by the Government of this scholarship money. A visit to us in the Easter vacation by a staff member of another similar school helped us to understand a little better the problems involved, but gave us little guidance as to how to avoid the same violence in our own college.

Letters were sent to Government officials at our local township and regional capital. Visits were made to two senior educational establishments in the area where scholarships had already been received. Gleaning all the information we could ahead of time, we prepared a document as to how we felt we should disburse the money when it came. Copies of this document were sent to the central Government in Kinshasa and also to church leaders, regional educational directors and local directors of other subsidized schools, to elicit their comments, corrections or criticisms. We received no response. No-one was willing to commit himself.

A Government conference in Kisangani on medical education enabled two of our staff to ask again for clear direction as to what we were expected to do when the cash arrived. Once again, there was no answer. Basically they would only say, rather cryptically: 'Wait until you have the cash: it may never come!'

Two members of this regional conference then flew up to

inspect our college at Nyankunde. I shall tell more of this inspection in a moment, but during it they had an unpremeditated meeting with the student body, when they were faced with the same question direct from the students. On being asked what I proposed to do, I produced the document that we had prepared, not without considerable trepidation, as it was not a Government document and we never quite knew how far we could go on our own initiative.

The inspectors read out the document, line by line, painstakingly explaining each phrase, as to how the monthly 10 Zaires (£8) for each second- and third-year student would be allocated, to housing, schooling, clothing, feeding, and finally 20% as pocket-money. After checking various figures against our annual accounts, the inspectors eventually said that they considered it an extremely good document, the allocation fair and reasonable: if they had any criticism, it was only that 20% was too high for pocket-money. The Government reckoned that this was the money needed for existence, and pocket-money should be provided by the students' families.

I let out my breath with relief: the students almost hissed.

The atmosphere was electric, and I felt embarrassed before our distinguished visitors. Later on, over coffee, I asked if we had permission to allocate the 20% as pocket-money, and they assured me that, as director, it was entirely left to my discretion what I did, particularly as it meant that I was still subsidizing their fees to that amount out of my personal money.

We went ahead on this authority, albeit verbal only, and prepared documents in detail for every month of the current year, for each student, in duplicate, ready for the day the cash arrived. We trusted that, when it actually arrived, the students would be so thrilled to get their 20% that they would drop their mutterings, particularly now that they had heard their own authorities say that we were being more generous than others!

At the beginning of May 1973 a radio call informed us of an important conference in Kisangani for all those involved in para-medical teaching, particularly arranged for national and foreign nurses. I had been ill earlier in the year and missed many lectures. It was therefore felt wisest that I should not go. I was also leaving the country soon, and it was obviously more sense for those who would be carrying on to hear all the advice given. So Vera Thiessen, an American sister tutor in charge of the class-room teaching of nursing arts, and Camille Djailo, the national supervisor of students on ward practice, were nominated to represent our college at the conference. We prepared our 'file' of school dossier, information, statistics and questions, briefed the two of them on all we wanted to know, and sent them off.

Then an urgent radio message three days later from Vera.

'They want to meet you, and are coming to Bunia tomorrow.'

'Who? Can you repeat that message, Vera?'

Nothing but crackles and static interference answered us: we could make out no more, but were left to guess at the inference. In fact, we *were* prepared. We had lived six years in a state of preparedness for this moment. All our files were up to date, our teaching material in order, our time-tables carefully balanced. School accounts and statistics were all ready for instant inspection. Nevertheless, there was a wild rush of activity, to polish and tidy and lay out everything available; to prepare beds and meals; to clean dormitories and iron uniforms. A sense of expectant excitement filled the air.

The next day I went to Bunia with one of our African staff members and met the inspectors, a lady sister tutor from Kinshasa and a man from the Ministry of Education in Kisangani. We chatted happily and freely on the journey back to Nyankunde, where we arrived in time for the midday meal, generously provided and graciously prepared by Dr Ruth Dix. Then the afternoon was given up to the inspection. We did not spend long on the buildings: they were obviously pleased and satisfied. We spent longer in the class-rooms and offices, in the laboratory and nursing arts' demonstration room. They asked many searching questions and listened carefully to our replies and explanations.

The blackboard layout of all time-table programming for each staff member and each student for the whole year, in a fairly complex double-entry eight-colour system that we had devised, drew the longest discussion, and they were obviously impressed. Accounts and book-keeping, lists and statistics honestly did not interest them, and only with difficulty did I persuade them to sign these for me as being satisfactory. We discussed in detail the balance of practical experience with class-room theory; different pedagogic methods and approaches; student–staff relationships; the place of Party political involvement, especially where the Saturday active participation in manual labour was concerned, for medical workers. In everything they were clearly satisfied.

The next morning they met informally with the students for an hour and invited us, the foreign staff, to be present as well. There was an obvious element of suspicion. The students felt that the inspectors had probably sold them to the white staff and that we, the white staff, had talked the inspectors into accepting our point of view, as though we had something ulterior to gain through this inspection. Both inspectors did all they could to dispel this attitude. They openly praised the school, staff and students, for the obvious achievements: buildings, curriculum, uniforms, esprit-de-corps, examination results. All spoke of success, which in turn revealed hard united effort.

'Are there any questions you would like to ask us?'

I drew in my breath and waited.

'Is it essential that we girls should be midwives?'

A moment's stunned silence. I had not prepared the lady inspector for this particular problem of women's lib. in our midst.

'Essential?' she parried. 'But no. If you wish to remain with your second-year training diploma in general nursing, and work in the hospital, of course you may. We offer you the privilege of continuing a third year in midwifery.'

'Why can't we study with the boys, as health officers?'

This went on relentlessly for twenty minutes, just as the staff had had it all year. The lady inspector refused to lose patience, nor did she use sarcasm, but she clearly stated exactly what we had so often repeated. It was a privilege for a girl to train as a midwife, but a girl health officer was not wanted by the population, and service to our people must be our guide.

Eventually the Educational Inspector swung the question,

and so a male student brought up next the vexed question of money.

'We hear there are to be scholarships, back-dated to January. How is the money to be handled, and by whom?'

Again the inspector replied with care and courtesy, examined in detail our prepared document, and agreed that what we had planned was exactly in line with Government policy except that we were being too generous to offer them 20% as pocket-money! The students were furious, certain that I had previously primed the inspectors, or bribed them into saying what I wanted said.

Despite the hour of rather unpleasant questioning, as it seemed to me, both inspectors were very impressed by everything, including our student/staff relationship! They were quite amazed that we were able to encourage some 60% of our graduates to go back to the rural areas when they finished their studies at the Centre, as most other schools found that only 10% were willing to leave the city life.

I remember, as I gave them mid-morning coffee before driving them back to Bunia for the midday plane, asking them hesitantly if we could know the final 'mark' that would be attached to our inspection report. We needed seven out of the available ten to become officially recognized. It was so important to us, I hardly dared to breathe as I awaited some response.

The man shrugged and spread his hands. 'What can we say, really?'

This left me still quite uncertain and on tenterhooks of anxiety. Had he any idea of the importance of that moment to me as the climax of twenty years' hard work?

'Listen,' said the sister tutor. 'You are the last of the forty-three schools in our vast country of this standard of para-medical education that we have inspected. We have already given two schools nine, so what can we give you except ten? There is just no comparison.'

I nearly fainted.

'Thank you,' I whispered. 'Thank you.' I was addressing them both, yet I was also addressing in my mind and heart all the staff and all the students, all the helpers and workers, all who had been involved. 'Thank You, God.'

Chapter 10 June 1973
Apparent rejection

It seemed that our immediate goal, Government recognition for the college, resulting in legal diplomas for the graduates, was almost achieved. I confess I was thrilled. For seven years I had been working for this. In fact, quite honestly, for twenty years we had been working towards recognition, even if not always at Nyankunde. We had asked the Government in 1966 to give us eight years to achieve the standards required in permanent buildings, course material and qualified personnel. Now, in only seven years, one year ahead of our proposed schedule, we were in sight of completion.

When Government-subsidized salaries arrived for the teaching staff in 1971, we really knew that our request for recognition would be granted, as it was inconceivable that they would pay us unless they were content with our methods.

When Government doctors were sent for the final oral examinations and were authorized to use the legal rubber stamp on our diplomas, we were even more certain of our ultimate acceptance.

When the inspectors had arrived and spoken so favourably, and shown us the copy of their report recommending 'immediate recognition, and speedy upgrading', it was obvious that it was only a matter of time before the coveted official document would arrive, recognizing us as a Government school for training national para-medical workers. Add to this the fact that the inspectors had brought with them the blank legal diplomas for us to fill in for each finalist student of that year, and our joy was full.

Monday, 26 June, only four weeks since the inspection and eleven days after the final oral examinations, dawned like any other day of our tropical year, at 5.30 a.m., bright and clear, with a mild haze over the distant hills. I went down the hill early to college as we had a lot of work to get through. The other staff soon joined me in the library, where we prepared for the day's activities.

Each student had a six-week summer holiday to visit his own people and to collect his fees for the coming school year. Half of each class would go on holiday from 27 June till 11 August, while the other half worked in the wards and outpatients' clinics of the hospital. A week of overlap from 11 to 18 August made allowance for transport difficulties, and also enabled us to arrange our 'Big Day' with the whole college together.

We were inviting the 1968 graduating class to come for an 'old-boys' reunion on 14 August. The 15th would be a welcome meeting for two new doctors, Philip and Nancy Wood, who were expected to arrive early in August to take over the direction of the college. In the afternoon there would be the presentation of the diplomas to the new graduating class. The 16th was to be a farewell meeting and evening party for me, as I felt that the time had come to leave Nyankunde and to hand over to younger workers.

Arrangements were well in hand. Transport had been arranged for all those hoping to come. Local Government officials had been invited to be with us and to share in the programme. The choir had been practising for five months. I hoped to have cassette recorders running throughout the three days and had acquired films for my camera, in order to have a permanent record of the final achievement of my twenty years' work in Africa. After the three days of festivities, at the end of the week, the second half of the student body, including all those finally leaving us at the end of their three years of study, would go for their holidays till the end of September. Those back from their homes would take over the hospital duties.

Before leaving for holiday, each student of the first group needed to receive his annual report card and class bulletin, a certificate in lieu of diploma, a road-pass and student identity card for claiming reduction of fares on public transport, and various other items, differing for each area and student. Usually we gave them their tickets if we had managed to secure these ahead of time, and some pocket-money to enable them to reach their homes without hardship. Added to this, each student needed to check the wording and spelling on his diploma which had to be sent to the Government for ratification and signature.

Besides all this, this year each senior student was to receive a bonus gift, as we thought of it, from the newly-arrived Government scholarship money. We had worked hard to decide how to allocate this money justly. The Government had sent almost £10 for each second- and third-year student for each month from January to July. When we completed the annual school accounts for 1 July 1972 to 30 June 1973, it was obvious that this £10 a month per student would barely cover the cost of feeding, clothing and schooling the students, let alone housing and administration. However, we felt we wanted them to have at least some of the money, as pocket-money, while we accepted the responsibility to continue a certain amount of subsidy.

Eventually we decided to give them 20% of the money for the six months January to June, and all the July allocation if they were on vacation. The 80% that we retained (for 35 students this came to about £1,500 at that moment) would enable us to prepare adequately for the coming school year, as the regional educational authority's gift had done the previous year. In future, the regular monthly income would help the college to run smoothly without being so dependent on foreign subsidies; doubtless this was the object of the Government's scholarship scheme. We had already prepared carefully-worded explanatory forms for each senior student for each of the seven months involved. Each student would be asked to sign in duplicate for each month's allocation.

At 7.0 a.m. the first three students came in together, all third-year students who were being invited to return after their vacation to join the staff for a year as hospital supervisors. They would be largely responsible for the training of first-year students in the art of nursing. Albert Amuli was one of these, and he showed every promise of being an excellent and capable leader in the future.

Basuana, Vera Thiessen and I had sorted out all the 'piles' of certificates, road-passes and money for each student. We explained things again carefully to these first three, getting them to check each document for signature, the correct date, the spelling of names: to check the road-passes and tickets for the correct destination. They knew the routine well from previous years. We then gave them a certain allocation of gift money, approximately the price of their journey home plus 50p for every night spent on the journey. Amuli lived six days' journey away to the south-west, almost 1,000 miles by road, and he received approximately £12 for this.

Then we explained again all that had been discussed four weeks previously when the inspectors had been with us, concerning the scholarship money. We showed them the duplicated receipt-forms and how the money was being used. We then offered them £22 each as pocket-money to take home, and asked them to sign for it.

Probably my own subconscious fear didn't help the situation. I knew it might not be smooth sailing, though I tried to carry it off with an easy optimism. I knew that there had been mutterings among the students ever since they had heard that scholarship money was coming. And even before that they had believed that, since the staff received Government salaries, there must have been money sent for them which I was not handing over. They simply couldn't believe that their Government would pay us, foreign staff, a salary without sending anything for them, the students. It mattered so much to me that all should go smoothly and without trouble. It mattered to me that they should trust me and not suspect that I was trying to cheat them or do them down. Instinctively we, the staff, knew that if these three senior students signed the rest would follow suit. I tried to will them to accept our word and sign their names.

They pulled the piles towards them. Painstakingly and slowly they went through each document, checking spellings, dates, signatures. They counted the money. They studied the receipt-forms. They made their own calculations. No-one spoke.

I tried to chatter nonchalantly, about their holidays, their families, our next year together on the staff and how much we were looking forward to having them back. I reminded them of our 'Big Day' and urged them to make every effort to start their return journey in time to be with us. All the time I was praying for them to sign.

We could feel the tension. They didn't look at each other. They didn't speak to each other. They listened to my patter – and I almost believed that they were going to sign.

'Please, please sign,' my heart was urging them. I feared whatever would happen if they refused. As always I was un-certain of my ground. I knew that what we were doing was in accordance with Government guide-lines. I knew that it was absolutely honest, and that the students were getting more, not less, than others would have given them. Yet if there was a show-down with Government officials called in, in the present climate of an African country, with feelings running high against white foreigners, the whole situation could very easily be turned against us.

They wouldn't sign.

Each had been meditatively chewing the tip of his ball-point pen, checking and re-checking each form. I felt that each one was waiting to see if one of the others would give in and sign. Slowly each one put down the pen and pushed the money back towards us. As I remember it, they said nothing. Their very silence was a bit uncanny and unnerving.

Carefully and patiently I went through all our reasoning again. I had the account books there and all the relevant Gov-ernment correspondence. I offered to show them anything they wanted to convince them that not only were we acting in ac-cordance with their own Government's wishes, but actually being generous over and above. Perhaps that was the mistake. The fact that we indicated that we could be generous to a cer-tain degree made them question our ultimate honesty in saying that we couldn't give them all the money.

Still they refused to sign.

I know I was beginning to feel desperate. These were our best students, both academically and also spiritually. If they could be convinced that it was right that they sign, that they were making a mistake to refuse, the rest of the student body would probably accept their lead without too much difficulty.

They offered no explanation, no reasoning. However, we knew instinctively that they had made up their minds to accept nothing less than 100% of the back-pay scholarship money to January, and that probably they would consent to pay school fees the next year out of what followed. These first three were all graduating, so there would be no 'future payment'. I guessed that as soon as they had heard, via the African grape-vine, that the money was coming, £10 each month for the past six months, they had already decided what they would buy – a new suit, a transistor radio or a bicycle. What we were offering, 20% of it, simply made these purchases impossible and they felt cheated.

Perhaps they tried to reason about the rightness of their attitude and the wrongness of mine, though they said nothing.

'You've already fed us for these six months, so why take the money now? It's the same with clothes and housing and schooling. Why are you asking us to pay you back what you've already given? If you wanted it back, why didn't you say so last January, that it was only a loan?'

But they maintained a rigid, stony silence.

We sent the three away and called in other students, one by one. With each one we had exactly the same situation. A careful perusal of everything, a silent reading and studying of the explanatory notes, an acceptance of all their papers and road-passes – but a complete refusal to sign for and accept the money.

After about three or four more students, we called a halt for breakfast. During the break we gathered the other members of staff together and told them what was happening. Together we prayed that God would break the deadlock. We were almost certain that this was some kind of *likilimba*, an agreement between them all, like a trade union strike, plus threats of brutality for anyone who 'gave in to the whites' and signed for and accepted their partial monies. It was a determined, concerted action by all of them to stand out for 'their rights', and to have the 100% of that back-pay scholarship money.

We decided to start again, and to call each of the three seniors separately and give them a chance to yield to our request without the direct hindrance of losing face in front of another. We promised that no-one should know who signed and who didn't. Apparently this was another wrong move and only hardened their resolve to resist our efforts. We were not exactly skilled in the art of strike-breaking, nor of conciliation between management and floor!

When Albert came in, he very nearly gave in to our earnest pleading and exhortation. He had been mission- and church-trained all his life, and all his school and college fees had been paid by his local church and missionaries. Deep in his heart, he knew he was throwing away something of lasting value by refusing to trust us. He took the pen from me and drew the form towards him. He read it all again and bent over it, poised to sign. Then suddenly, abruptly, he pushed it from him and said: 'No, no, I can't.' Looking up at me, he continued in a self-defensive, almost pathetic whisper: 'What's the good of *one* signing, anyway?' and with this cryptic remark he rushed from the room.

We sensed, rather than understood, that fear had ruled him, a fear which perhaps we staff could barely appreciate. He knew what awaited him outside if he broke the oath that they had taken together to refuse to accept our terms, and he just couldn't face the consequences. It was no good my telling him that no-one need know. He knew that they would know at once when he joined them: he just couldn't bluff them all. And he was deeply afraid.

Throughout that Monday we saw, individually, each of the students due for the first holiday shift. We treated each one similarly, patiently, prayerfully. We refused to accept the situation. We prayed earnestly for a crack, that perhaps just one would have the courage of his convictions and stand out against the crowd. We had no real idea of what might be involved in the 'oath of allegiance' or of the threats employed by the ring-leaders.

Girl students were also being asked to sign a request-form to return to do midwifery studies in their third year, instead of public health studies as the male students did. In asking this, we had known that we were throwing down a gauntlet. Only one second-year girl student out of the four, though five first-year students out of the six, signed willingly, and then she pleaded with us not to let the others know that she had signed. This gave us even greater certainty that strong threats were being employed by the directors of the revolt.

On Tuesday we started all over again. We asked Dr Becker to come and speak to the assembled college, to explain that what we were doing was absolutely in accord with the directions from their own leaders in Government authority; and that either they signed and accepted the money they were being offered, or else they could go home without the money, which would be returned to the Government. We were not free to choose what we would do with it: it belonged to the Government. Obviously we could not hold the money, even though it was sent for college funds, unless the students signed for it, as the Government receipt-forms were all made out in each individual's name.

We spent another seemingly long day, re-interviewing each student. We refused to give in half-way: we felt each one must be given the opportunity in private to change his mind following Dr Becker's words. No-one changed his mind. No-one signed his receipt-form.

I went to bed at midnight on Tuesday with a very heavy heart. I had discussed the situation carefully with our African members of staff, and with Africans in the local education offices. They all advised us to stick to what we had said, though they were obviously becoming nervous. If the students went to report the situation to local 'Party' headquarters, nobody was quite sure how the situation would look to an outsider. My heaviness of heart was not only caused by the impasse we were in, but also because these were *our* students. I loved them. I cared for them. For three years I had taught the seniors, preparing them for their future life-service, as medical evangelists in the service of the church and their fellow countrymen. They were like sons to me. Now I felt that they had turned on me, at the last moment – the moment of our apparent triumph with Government recognition. Later, when I heard them arraign me publicly, I really felt that they had rejected me, but already I sensed their almost-callous spurning. They appeared to have put up with me, my leadership, my administration and all the work we had slaved to do on their behalf to get the recognition;

but now that it had come, they didn't want us any more. They wanted to show their independence of us. Even worse, I sensed that they didn't really trust us. All our reasoning was just words to them, easy words from the white foreigner to show once more how good and generous we were. It was as though all the daily radio brain-washing to beware of the deceit of the 'hated imperialist westerner' was suddenly bursting into fruit. They believed it, and so they did not believe us.

On Wednesday morning Dr Becker rang me and asked me to go down the hill to see him. By now the whole college was involved, not just the half going on vacation. All but ten of the first-year students were on strike. There was hardly a student nurse in the whole 250-bed hospital nor any to help with the thousand outpatients. Everybody at the Centre knew of the deadlock, and they were all watching closely.

'All right,' Dr Becker said to me as I entered his little office. 'We'll have the committee at six this evening.'

Uncertainly I looked at him for some explanation.

'I beg your pardon, Sir?' I queried.

'The committee can meet this evening,' he repeated, looking at me with obvious sorrow in his eyes.

'I don't quite understand, Sir. Which committee?'

He now looked puzzled and pushed a letter towards me.

'But you have asked for the executive committee to take over and sort out the problem in the college.' He spoke quietly, but there was a mild reproachfulness in his tone, at what must have seemed to him my deliberate obtuseness,

I picked up the letter, a piece of college note-paper, and read the short line of request for the executive committee to take over 'as we are unable to reach an acceptable solution', and then I read the several signatures. Dr Becker had not noticed that mine was not among them.

A lump rose in my throat. So my own staff felt I couldn't cope. I suppose I was unreasonable in my sheer weariness with the affair, but I felt that not only the students, but now also the staff had rejected my leadership. Doubtless this wasn't true in the slightest, but I was touchy. I guess that I was proud of being a good and fair and competent leader. I had led a para-medical training school all my twenty years in Congo/Zaire, and felt I really knew how to cope and handle affairs on all levels. And this was my last term, my last chance in a sense to show my colours. I didn't stop to think, or to ask the staff why they had taken this step. I had been ill only four months previously and this was probably a considerate action in order to save me too much involvement in sorting out the strike: but it just didn't register like that to me at that moment.

'O.K., Sir. I'll see everything is ready,' I answered Dr Becker politely, as I stumbled almost blindly from his office, wrapped in my own wounded feelings.

The day was spent preparing. There was a lot to do. All members of an extended executive committee had to be notified, including members of the local education office as they were closely involved with the college, particularly where finance was concerned. Certain local church elders were also invited, as the affair might well develop into a disciplinary one.

The annual financial statement was rushed through, simplified, duplicated and made available in French and in Swahili for each committee member to examine and to compare with the statistical reasoning involved in the employment of the scholarship money. All this was also carefully laid out and explained on the large blackboards in diagrammatic form. A brief concise history of the application for the scholarship money was compiled, and copies made available of all the correspondence of the previous six months as it related to the affair in hand.

At six o'clock everyone assembled, but they immediately rearranged the room from usual committee procedure, to resemble a law-court. Dr Becker took the chair and I was asked to sit on his right. Then three representative students were allowed to enter, to present their case against me.

It was unbelievable, really. To me it was the climax of twenty years of service. If I hadn't been leaving Africa in three months' time, I might have been able to look at things a little less passionately, a little more objectively. But, nevertheless, the shock of hearing my own students give a carefully-prepared, reasoned attack on me would have been humiliating at any time. I was basically accused of stealing college funds. They reasoned that, since the staff were subsidized, this proved that

174

the college was recognized and that therefore we had been receiving student subsidies from the same date. That I had continued to demand £50 per annum per student, despite receiving Government grants, was plainly stealing. I was accused of lying, in denying these facts; of duplicity in being able to argue my way out of the situation every time it had been approached. They also stated that I had falsified the accounts and report-sheets sent to the Government so that they would not know that I was systematically misappropriating college funds.

The whole, long, twenty-minute tirade was recorded on cassette. It sounded even worse when I listened to it again the next day. The final cruelty was that the chosen spokesman for the students was Albert Amuli, our senior student, a man brought up in our own church schools and whose school fees had been consistently paid by church and missionaries.

By midnight we had achieved nothing. Much abuse had flowed. Mud was flung at many others besides myself, particularly anyone who tried to reason with them or show them how stupid they were being. We all separated and went to our various homes wearied, dispirited, discouraged. I couldn't sleep. I just felt utterly dejected, with a growing sense of personal failure.

I picked up my Bible and sought God's guidance. It didn't come easily. I prayed, but felt as though I was talking to myself, or, at best, to the ceiling. I wept, mostly out of self-pity. I tried the Bible again, re-reading the passage for my next day's regular reading, straight through the four chapters of the book of Jonah. I seemed to get nothing from it at all, no consolation, no strength, no guidance. I cried out in desperation to God to give me something to meet my need. I read Jonah for the third time that night, and began to see some sense.

The storm that shook Jonah awake, that upset a vast crowd of people, the sailors, passengers, those who sent cargo, those who were waiting to receive the cargo, other ships with their crews and passengers and cargo in the immediate vicinity, was all because God wanted to speak to one man, Jonah. When he jumped overboard the storm stopped, the ship reached its destination, and there is no particular indication that anyone

175

was permanently affected. The sailors made a passing act of acknowledgment of the power of this God of Jonah by the offering of a sacrifice of appeasement: that was all.

'O.K., Lord, you want to speak to *me*, and my deaf ears have caused this storm in which everyone – all the students and staff of the college and medical centre, all the 250-bed patients and over one thousand outpatients – is becoming involved. O.K., I'll jump overboard – then what?'

So I wrote a letter of resignation as college director and sent it down to Dr Becker for the executive committee early the next morning. Probably, deep down in my heart, I didn't expect such a letter to be accepted, even though I had specifically asked that no-one question it. Wasn't I indispensable to them? How could they run and handle the college without me? So my heart reasoned, hoping against hope that they would refuse to accept my resignation.

They accepted my letter, presumably gratefully. I chewed my heart out in private chagrin and allowed my self-pity to make an enormous mountain out of the rapidly growing ant-hill. Not only students and staff, but now fellow committee members were glad to get on without me.

My house help, Benjamin, kept me in touch with events. All the second- and third-year students were sent home, having received 80% of their scholarship money, the college retaining 20%, all receipts having been duly signed. They were not to be invited to return unless they apologized for their behaviour and language, accepted a period of discipline from their local churches for having involved patients in their strike action, and signed a statement with regard to the allocation of future scholarship money.

They left on Saturday. Not one came to say good-bye or to shake hands. There were no photos of this qualifying class, my last group of students. There was to be no diploma day. All August festivities were to be cancelled – including the choir, despite five months of hard practising, and no recordings to take home. I went into Bunia, to give a report to the Government education office, as we were directly responsible to them. I had to tell them and Dr Biki that there would be no graduation day celebrations as previously planned, to which they had already been invited. I felt very small. I wrote to the regional inspector of education at Kisangani, who had become a personal friend over the last two or three years and who had also been invited to our diploma day, both to represent the Party and also to present the diplomas. I told him briefly of the recent events and the reason for the cancellation of our graduation celebrations. By then, my pride was truly laid in the dust and trampled upon.

'Is it really worth while?'

The niggling question that I wouldn't look at, that I didn't want to hear, kept pressing up into the level of conscious thought.

'O.K. Right now, after all your philosophizing and encouraging others, just answer: has it all been worth it?'

Chapter 11 September 1973
Was it all worth while?

The question had to be answered, I knew, and it really must be answered in Africa before I left, but for a few weeks I couldn't bring myself to face it squarely.

I knew of course that the staff and committee had not really rejected me. As I have said, I had been in hospital only four months earlier with complete nervous exhaustion after six months of intense activity. During that time I had had to make three trips from Nyankunde to Ibambi and Nebobongo, two by lorry, involving twenty or more hours of hard driving in each direction. Each trip had involved emotional, medical and spiritual commitments. The first had been for the triumphant funeral of our field leader, Jack Scholes, whom I had loved as a father through eighteen years of co-operation; the second had been for the Christmas and New Year conferences of church and mission, probably my last in Africa; and the third had been with regard to establishing our church medical services within the new Government framework of a national service, with the tremendous amount of documentation needed.

Apart from these journeys there was all the routine work of the college, with more than twenty hours a week in the classroom, preparation for classes, marking of test papers, keeping of student report-files and general college administration. Again, special extra work was being put in preparatory to handing over the leadership of the college to the two new doctors. Add to all this the growing tensions of a changing political climate, with increasing uncertainty as to the popularity of the white foreigner on African soil, and the scene had been well set for some sort of physical reaction. There was a limit, I suppose, beyond which I had just no right to push my body to keep up with my more ambitious mind and spirit; but I hadn't heeded the warning light. So a week in hospital had been essential, followed by four weeks of slow convalescence in the home of one of our kindly American nurses at the centre.

With this in their minds, it was hardly surprising that the team felt that they ought not to allow me to try to carry the load alone when the strike started. In fact, it would have been extremely surprising if they had sat back and left me to cope! It wasn't as if the college was mine (even though the way I spoke and acted might indicate that I thought it was): it was part of the whole medical centre, and we were all involved.

The staff knew my peculiarly stubborn streak, and that my pride would not let me give in to student pressure to lower the standard, as I saw it. Yet they could also see that there was another side to the problem. Looked at through African eyes, things were often not as clear-cut as they seemed to us foreigners. True, the scholarship money was given for the running of the college, but then the college had run for the past six months. The students had been fed from January to June and the food paid for, so why take the money for that now? They were clothed, and the tailors' salaries had all been paid, so why take money for that?

I was allowing myself to think that they, the staff and committee, had compromised by giving in to the students' blackmail: 'We'll report you to Party headquarters if you don't. . . .' And yet, deep down, I knew this couldn't be so. They had clearly felt that a difference could and should be made between back-pay and future scholarship moneys. An agreement had been reached between management and workers, financially acceptable to both. To us, as college administrators, this was obviously unsatisfactory, as we had to plan ahead: get in stocks of food, books, cloth; prepare a budget for the coming year – and Government subsidies were notoriously unreliable. Yet through the previous seven years here at Nyankunde, God had never failed to provide all our needs. Couldn't He continue to do so? Did the coming of Government subsidies change our reliance on God as sole provider for our daily needs? If so, we would need to look closely as to the underlying motive in the seven-year struggle to obtain recognition.

Then I had to realize that the students were *not* mine. How they would have resented my thinking of them in this way! Student involvement should only have been a small part of my total involvement in the local church situation. These particular students were only a very few out of the two hundred and more who had passed through the college.

Living went on. The routine responsibility of the end of another college year, with all the Government forms to be completed and sent off by a certain prescribed date, kept me busy and occupied. The continued preparation for the arrival of Philip and Nancy Wood, both in the home and also in the school, filled most of my spare moments so that I hadn't too much time for morbid introspection. I had the opportunity to spend two weeks away from Nyankunde, at a neighbouring Christian village in the mountains with missionary friends, being much spoilt, and this did a lot to restore balance and perspective.

The Lord reminded me sharply of that traumatic night of 29 October 1964, and how I had gone home on furlough in 1965 and testified all over the United Kingdom to His sufficiency. It had been true. On that dreadful night, beaten and bruised, terrified and tormented, unutterably alone, I had felt at last that even God had failed me. Surely He could have stepped in earlier, surely things need not have gone that far. I had reached what seemed to me the ultimate depth of despairing nothingness. Yet even as my heart had cried out against God for His failure and my mental anguish taunted me to doubt His very existence, another reasoning had made itself felt.

'You asked Me, when you were first converted, for the privilege of being a missionary. This is it: don't you want it?'

Events had moved so fast: everything seemed to happen at once. Pain and cruelty and humiliation had continued in an ever-growing crescendo, yet with it, a strange peace and deep consciousness that God *was* in charge and knew what He was doing. Odd thoughts and phrases and impulses broke through, and later on were woven together to show the inner meaning of the events of that night, but it had not been orderly, in a way one could set down on paper or explain in a lecture.

'These are not your sufferings: they are Mine. All I ask of you is the loan of your body.'

Again the overwhelming sense of privilege, that Almighty God should stoop to ask of me, a mere nobody in a forest clearing in the jungles of Africa, something He needed. They had called Him 'a worm, no man'. I said I wanted to be identified with Him, yet did I really want to be a worm, trodden on, spurned, ignored? No! Yet this was the privilege He offered, the privilege of being a missionary, His ambassador, identified with Him among those whom He wanted to serve.

'You went home and told everyone that I was sufficient at *that* moment, in *those* circumstances. Isn't this true now, in today's circumstances?'

I tried to say: 'But of course, Lord. You know it's true.'

'No,' He quietly rebuked me. 'No. You no longer want Jesus only, but Jesus plus ... plus respect, popularity, public opinion, success and pride. You wanted to go out with all the trumpets blaring, from a farewell-do that you organized for yourself: with photographs and tape-recordings to show and play at home, just to reveal what *you* had achieved. You wanted to feel needed and respected. You wanted the other missionaries to be worried about how ever they'll carry on after you've gone. You'd like letters when you got home to tell you how much they realize they owe to you, how much they miss you. All this and more. Jesus *plus* ... No, you can't have it. Either it must be "Jesus only" or you'll find you've no Jesus. You'll substitute Helen Roseveare.'

A great long silence followed – several days of total inner silence. At last I managed to tell Him that with all my heart I wanted 'Jesus only'.

I went back to Nyankunde, sobered and humbled, and completed preparations for Philip and Nancy's arrival. They flew into Bunia airport early on Monday morning, 13 August 1973. It really was marvellous to welcome them and drive them out to Nyankunde, watching them drinking in the beauty of our hills and views across the valley. The tempo of events really speeded up now, as we had only six weeks together before I was due to leave for the United Kingdom: six short weeks in which to hand over, in orderly fashion, what it had taken twenty years to create, and in which they were also to learn as much as possible of the Swahili language.

After three days locally, meeting everyone, seeing over the Nyankunde village, getting a quick bird's-eye view of the whole, collecting the necessary residence cards, opening a bank account and acquiring driving licences, we set off to drive to Ibambi and Nebobongo. It seemed right to introduce them the hard way to African transport problems! Within the first fifty miles we met our first major mudhole with an 8-ton lorry firmly entrenched across the narrow, one-track road. Surrounding crowds lined the route and watched interestedly. No-one offered a hand, but everyone offered advice. A local church group pushed us through and enabled us to reach our immediate destination only two hours late. On Friday, the second day of our trip, the 300 miles took from 4.30 a.m. to 11.30 p.m. and involved the negotiation of some ten mud-holes of varying intensity, length and depth, but of unvarying nerve-racking interest.

Saturday we spent at Ibambi, meeting missionaries and national church leaders, and welcoming Nancy and Philip into the family. On Sunday we went to a local church, some 30 miles north-east of Ibambi, and spent a wonderful day with over 1,000 local Christians, gathered under a palm-frond shelter and overflowing it in every direction, worshipping God. The singing was whole-heartedly African. The crowd ebbed and flowed; children trotted in and out; chickens and goats wandered around unhindered and unnoticed. The sun beat down. Older men tended to doze after noon in their deck-chairs, till a rousing hymn jerked them back into active participation. Different groups of children or women or youth took part with specially-prepared items. Several different speakers, using any one of the three main languages of the area, took turns in exhorting the crowd. There was no formal direction to the service, and yet all was obviously controlled and orderly. It certainly was an experience for anyone's first Sunday in the tribal areas of inner Africa.

On Monday we started our week at Nebobongo, the first of

many for Philip, my last after twenty years of 'belonging'. Eleven of our para-medical workers had gathered, from as far afield as Malingwia, 250 miles to the north-west, and Opienge, the same distance to the south. The workers had cycled in, some taking as much as five days to reach us. This was their welcome to their two new doctors; it was a week of refreshment, medically and spiritually, with daily teaching sessions and demonstrations; and it was to be their farewell to me.

Each day was full and varied. It was obvious from the start that we would not achieve all that we had planned, but we did our best. The pervading spirit of joy and harmony made work a pleasure. The whole team pulled together. The desire to learn and profit from the week was in evidence right from the start: everyone put all they had into it, to make it a great success. I was tremendously happy. These were my people: I was one of them, accepted by them. Each day the soreness grew at the thought of tearing oneself away, leaving them, and starting to make a new life again elsewhere.

Particularly was this so where John Mangadima was concerned. For twenty years we had worked together. Of course there had been ups and downs, times when he maddened me, times when I irritated him, even times when we doubted and distrusted each other: but we'd come through, and were now very closely knit in spirit. My deepest joy in leaving was to know that John was appointed as assistant medical director to Philip Wood, for the running and supervision of our medical services in our church area. I had prayed and worked so hard for that. He had a Yamaha motorcycle to enable him to visit all our hospitals and dispensaries regularly, and I couldn't suppress a grin as I watched him setting off to Ibambi, with all the aplomb of one who had owned it all his life.

One afternoon, as he and Philip were operating together in the theatre, I had entered his office to glean a few facts before coming home. He had come in while I was there, peeling off his surgical gloves.

'Hi, Doctor. What are you doing in here?'

'Oh, just copying down a few facts and figures to tell folk back home.'

He leant over my shoulder and saw the last line I had

written: 372 major operations in 1972 with only six surgical deaths.

'Oh, Doctor, don't bother with things like that. Just tell them that nearly 200 people found Christ as their Saviour through the medical services last year.'

I turned and hugged him, my eyes filling with tears of joy. And God said pretty plainly: 'Isn't My way better than yours?'

The journey back to Nyankunde the following Monday was more cruel than usual. At 5.30 p.m., after an extremely good thirteen hours of driving, we came upon the king of mud-holes, 400 yards of a churned-up sea of mud, at some places more than 6 feet deep, already with several large transport-lorries involved. It was 3.30 a.m. when Philip and Basuana eventually struggled through, to join Nancy and myself at a small village up the next hill. We'd gone ahead on foot, to dry out and rest after the first gruelling five hours of effort. We eventually dragged wearily into Nyankunde at midday, ready to start straight into a new school year the next week.

It was a little strange, as the first Monday morning in September dawned, when Philip and Nancy went down the hill to college at 6.30 a.m. and I realized that I really had handed over. It was theirs now, not mine. There were still many ways to help them in the remaining three weeks, particularly in the office and in language-study. We made the most of every available hour.

Suddenly my last week-end was on me and I could hardly bear to consider all that was involved. On the Friday, the missionary family had arranged a farewell party for me. It was very touching. All my special African friends were there, as well as all the missionaries. Speeches were made. I felt choked and too full up to say much, and I knew it was sincere and not just laid on for the occasion.

On Saturday afternoon the Africans had a party for me down at the college. When I arrived at five o'clock and was led through the waiting crowd to the top table, I glanced round and saw all my friends of the past seven years, masons and plumbers, tailors and cooks, office workers and teaching staff, church elders and choir members, printers from the local press and gardeners from the school allotments. My eyes filled with tears as I sensed the love in their welcome to me.

A goat had been cooking over a spit for the past twenty-four hours, and Philip duly carved it. Food poured in, in steaming dishes and bowls from the kitchen, served by first-year students. Chatter was soon flowing in the usual free, happy way of Africa as everyone ate their fill. Two ludicrous skits followed from staff members and brought roars of laughter. Then the small group of third-year students who had returned after all the sadness of June, and who had asked to be taken back into college, had sung for me words they had written themselves, basically asking me to remember them as my sons who loved me, and to let God blot out from my memory the sore wound they had tried to inflict on me in their stupidity. Again, my heart was strangely moved and touched.

Philip made a short speech in Swahili, his first public usage of the language, much to everyone's delight, thanking me for all the service to the college over the past seven years. By then I had scribbled down all the thoughts that I wanted to express to everyone, in groups and individually, to say thank you to them for all their love and friendship over the years.

'Now it is over to you,' Philip concluded, addressing the more than sixty African guests. 'If you have anything you want to say, now is your chance.' Turning to me, he added in English: 'Not you; you just wait a bit.'

Then they started. For two hours it went on. I don't know how many spoke, probably more than twenty of them. I don't remember much of what was said. I cried: it was very, very moving. One I remember especially, but many others were like him: Nyelongo, our mason.

'You don't remember, Doctor, but one day when we were building the main school block I was late for work. I was scared: roll-call was over and you had already gone into school. When you came out at eight o'clock you came straight over to me and asked how my baby was. I didn't even know that you knew I had a baby!

' "The baby is very sick," I told you.

' "Where is the baby?" you asked.

' "Back at home."

' "But why not in the hospital?" and you sounded irritated.

' "We can't afford the hospital card and care," I replied.

'Then you really were mad! You went straight up the hill to your home, got into your Land Rover, came charging down on to the building site and shouted to me to get in. I'd never been in a car before. You told me to direct you to our village, but no car had ever been to our village before. You didn't seem to care, and we went, jolting and bumping over the mountain-side. I called my wife and collected the baby, and you took us all to the hospital.'

I guess his child must have been very ill, as he said I told him not to return to work till we saw whether his child would live. He probably missed three or four days' work. He continued his story:

'At the end of the month, I came with the rest to be paid. I was trying to pluck up courage to ask you to spread my debt over several months, rather than take my whole month's pay. When you called my name, you passed me my wage-packet like everyone else. I just stared at you in unbelief. Then I rushed round the side of the house, laid the money out on the ground and counted it. It was all there.

'I ran all the way home. I called my wife. "Look, look, our money is all here. She hasn't taken *any* off, not even for the days' work I missed, let alone for our baby's care and treatment."

'We cried. Then we knelt down, and we suddenly realized all that you and Basuana meant when you told us day after day of God's love: and we asked God then and there into our hearts and lives and have followed Him ever since.'

I drew a deep breath as he sat down. I was deeply stirred. I wouldn't be surprised if, when I made up the wage-packets that month long ago, I had simply forgotten that Nyelongo owed money! I'm like that. But God had not forgotten. He used that little, almost insignificant, event in our daily relationship: not through a Sunday preaching engagement, but just an ordinary work job; and He had brought about His purposes, and I had merely been one of the links in the chain. This was it. This was what Evangelist Agoya had said to me years ago at Nebobongo; it was what Basuana had said to me much more recently here at Nyankunde: 'We can't all be the last link in the chain.' Being the last link may bring public acclaim and a sort of popularity: but being willing to be any link, however inconspicuous, brings happiness and lasting joy.

The question returned in my heart: 'Has it all been worth while?'

As others testified, my mind strayed round the north-eastern region of Zaire to our many regional hospitals and rural dispensaries. I pictured our many graduates working singly or in pairs, in far-off places, putting into practice all we had taught them. I began to count them, mentally ticking them off on a list. Tokpo and Ezo at Malingwia; Balani at Poko and the lovely small hospital he had built himself, loved and respected by everyone; Anizanga at Nala, Angola at Gamba. There was Jacqueline van Bever at Betongwe doing an excellent job; Sengi at Ibambi, Boloki at Buambi and Tahilo at Opienge. Then of course at Nebobongo, the whole team with John Mangadima, Asea, Namuniabangi and Bundayi. Way down to the south, Basetea had gone with his wife and children as a missionary nurse to another tribal area and culture. Each name conjured up a face and a story. I could think of each one through his schooling, his problems and difficulties, his first job after graduating, his settling down and now becoming a really valuable member of the medical team. Many had had their teething troubles; some had had to undergo fairly severe church discipline; but they had come back the stronger and more reliable. There were so many of them. Not only those in our own church area, but in each of the various church regions: Ngonda at Aba, Rabama at Todro, Kasereka and others at Oicha, Mukwesi and others farther south in the Ruanguba area, Mandro doing dentistry at Itendeyi.

My heart thrilled as I continued to tick them off. There were the two whom we felt were called and set apart as future staff members for our training college, whom we had been able to send for further education, Mandaboy to be a nursing tutor, and Madrato possibly to be a doctor if he could procure a place at university.

Then I remembered so many others who weren't nurses or

medical workers, but who had been very much in the team since the beginning. Basuana had been such a good, close friend through nearly twenty years; Benj Gandisi the same. Church elders and pastors everywhere – Ndugu and Tamoma, Agoya and Taadi, too many to name – had become such close friends that I never even thought of them as black or any other colour. They were just those I loved, and I realized, as perhaps never before, just how much I loved them and was going to miss them when I left and went back to Britain.

The evening drew to a close. I wended my way up the hill to my little home, as Philip and Nancy drove some of the folk back to their homes, and I suddenly knew with every fibre of my being that these twenty years *had* been worth while, very, very worth while, utterly worth while, with no room left for regrets or recriminations.